Becoming *'You'*

FOR WOMEN

A Step-by-Step Guide to
**Self-Discovery
& Whole Self
Transformation**

Wendy Turner-Larsen MA MS MA

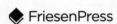 FriesenPress

Suite 300 - 990 Fort St
Victoria, BC, V8V 3K2
Canada

www.friesenpress.com

The recommendations within do not include any medical advice, medical interventions, or diagnosis of any kind. For medical advice, consult your health care professional. For psychological or mental health support, consult a registered psychologist or professional counsellor.

ISBN
978-1-5255-8674-3 (Hardcover)
978-1-5255-8673-6 (Paperback)
978-1-5255-8675-0 (eBook)

1. Self-Help, Personal Growth, Happiness

Distributed to the trade by The Ingram Book Company

"To find this level of profound healing within the cover of a single book is cause for celebration. The work inside personalizes and deepens with the addition of the written exercises to explore authentic self. A modern handbook for a truly individual journey for women."

—Janet, LCSW, MT USA

"*Becoming 'You' for Women* is written for both curious seekers and seasoned soul-searchers. This delightful and inspiring book provides a suite of personal and professional strategies to deal with the self-imposed barriers that often keep women from living their best life. Wendy Turner-Larsen is a subject area expert whose work assists women to become better acquainted with themselves by exploring their stories and removing the self-imposed barriers that no longer serve them. Now, her wisdom is captured in a clear, succinct and practical guide. I will be gifting this book over and over."

—Christina, Leadership Consultant, MA Leadership, BC Canada

"A must read. This is by far the best personal growth book I have ever come across. It is an excellent guide for both professional and personal growth that will lead you to discover and to love who you truly are."

—Michelle, Hypnotherapist, SK Canada

"There are lots of books out there that do a lot of 'telling', Wendy Turner-Larsen's book goes beyond the theory and takes you through a practical step by step process to get you were you want to 'be'. It is set up in an exceptional way to engage with other women as you work your way through the book and experience a very powerful, life changing journey."

—Lori, Leadership Coach & HR Consultant, MHRM, Human Resource Management, SK Canada

"I wish I'd read *Becoming* 'You' *for Women* earlier in life! Wendy Turner-Larsen has captured many of the issues I have battled as an adult woman, wife, mother and professional. *Becoming* 'You' outlines challenges such as people-pleasing, perfectionism and over-achievement, using the allegory of Sisyphus from Greek mythology and personal examples. The power of the stories lends credence to the powerful practical actions Turner-Larsen suggests. An excellent and easy read, this book may be viewed in its entirety or worked through in sections, on your own or in a group of women. Now that I have *Becoming* 'You' on hand, I can easily reread and remind myself that I do have everything I need within to become ME!"

—Sherri, Leadership Coach, Educator and Consultant, MEd, SK Canada

"Wendy invites you to learn more about yourself and provides the practical tools to assist you in *becoming* who you truly are."

—Candace, Professional Coach, SK Canada

Dedication

This book is dedicated to my husband, whose quiet, yet strong support has not only helped me complete this book but has helped me *become* who I really am.

This book is dedicated to all the women in my life. From each of you I have learned about *un* becoming and becoming.

Table of Contents

Section One

Un Becoming and Becoming
Why Is This Important?

Introduction

Un Becoming to Become You

Un becoming the 'you' you've created
to become who you really are.
You are enough. This is the new way.

"We cannot become what we need to be by remaining what we are."
—Max de Pree

I magine a world where women are powerful and strong. A world where women know they are enough, and they live and serve from that full *enough*-ness. A world where women live with the freedom to be who they really are. Imagine what women's lives could be, what families, communities, and organizations could be—what the *world* could be.

What if you were enough and truly believed it? What could be possible for you?

Becoming 'You' is your story about '*un* becoming' the person you've *created*. *Un* becoming allows who you *really* are to emerge: someone who truly knows and believes she is enough. You have everything it takes to undertake this metamorphosis. Within you, there is a vast reservoir of knowing, insight, and courage waiting to be harnessed.

Women have unique needs and challenges. We're wired and socialized to connect, and we often find ourselves over-doing, and over-focusing on others. This is part of the process that leads us to lose track of who we really are.

Popular culture encourages women to not be themselves, to set aside their hopes and dreams in service of the people around them. This sets us up for a unique set of psychological, emotional, and behavioural challenges; as we try to overcome them, we often end up trying to do it all, without the understanding, tools, or behaviours required to take care of our own fundamental needs. The opportunities exist for women to become CEOs and entrepreneurs, but society hasn't shifted to support this transition. We become tired, discouraged, and some of us never pause to determine how to do things differently. We burn out. This book is for women because women often focus externally on their family, friends, jobs, and communities. We push to do what needs to be done without full attention to ourselves, first. **At the core of this book** is the truth that you have everything you need to change whatever you *want* to change within yourself. For this to happen, you need to learn to trust yourself—your deeper knowing, your intuition, as this trust is essential for healthy living and becoming the real you. Many societal beliefs, pressures, and expectations (particularly our own) squash our trust in ourselves. Women struggle with this. Too often, we give our power away. We tend to wrestle with full acceptance of who we are: our gifts, talents, and greatness. Too many of us feel like we've got a hole in our beings which can never be filled. So, we desperately try to fill the hole, with external acceptance, affirmation, and doing.

We try to control ourselves. We try to control others. We try to control love. We try to control our success. We are left exhausted and empty.

As women we are inundated with messages of needing to be fixed. "Be more," we are told, "be better" and we buy into this.

We don't need to be fixed. We can know our own value! If you do this work and allow yourself to *un* become, you can become who you *really* are. You can not only feel happy and whole, emotionally and psychologically, but you can also find and flow with your life's purpose.

We need an emotionally safe place, just for women, where we can become who we really are. With the busyness, the expectations, the be-more and do-more push from society and ourselves, our connection to ourselves and other women is diminished. But we need to do this work in community.

This book is for you as a woman, because despite your external efforts, you know there is more for you. Not more *to do*, but more *to be*. Your first and most important relationship is with yourself.

This book is about *un becoming* to *become*, and we must recognize from the outset that this process never stops. You will never stop growing, deepening, seeing more fragmented pieces of yourself, healing yourself. Know that as you *un* become and unravel what is not you, you will become more of who you really are. You don't *un* become and *then* become. Both are always happening simultaneously.

These concepts are embedded in me through years of learning and practice. They have become the foundation of my life personally, and they can become yours too.

This is a woman's manual for full, life-long living. Approach this book however you want, in whatever way works for you. Skim through it, skip around, and read what resonates for you, depending on where you are in your life. You may decide to devote six months or a year of your life on the *un* becoming section. There is more information there than you need in any single 'work through', so you can come back again and again to certain sections, questions, writing prompts, and exercises that may resonate with you later. Although there is no 'right' way to read this book, I do recommend that at some point, you work with one chapter at a time, while reading, reflecting, journaling, and then creating some actions based on your learning. As you work through a section, try to create some space and time to shift and change, and then reflect and review on the process. And always remember: *you are enough.*

This process is a journey into deeper understanding, a journey to help you explore the deeper parts of yourself, to discover and uncover "you," and all the beauty your *you*-ness brings. *Un* becoming moves you out of a world of pushing against yourself and the world and into a world of living and being.

Diving In: *Un* Becoming to Become *You*, for Women

In Greek Mythology, there is a story about a King named Sisyphus. He lived a colourful life full of envy, strife, murder, and thievery—among other things. He usually got his way, until death came. Sisyphus attempted to avoid death by lying to the Gods. One of the Gods found out about his lies and manipulations, and as punishment, they condemned Sisyphus to an eternity in the underworld. He would push a rock up a hill only to have it fall back on him, every time. Every. Single. Time.

The moral I took from the story is this: we all get to a point in life when we realize we just can't keep pushing. Most of us don't behave the way Sisyphus did in his life, but we all get stuck in self-destructive beliefs that cause us to 'push'.

It's time to face the truth: the old way just won't get us the life we desire. We need a new way.

The rock Sisyphus was pushing was heavy because he still practiced his old ways of thinking and behaving. He continued to do what he had always done: push. But pushing will not get you the life you desire. That is the old way.

My personal journey has been one of pushing, and I continually meet clients cycling through this same pattern. Learning how to unravel my beliefs and get out of my own way has allowed me to *un* become, and now I feel called to share this journey with a wider audience. Pushing became a pattern for me. I pushed hard to succeed and to please. I pushed against myself, doing great damage to my spirit, my mind, and my physical health. The worst was when I hit the wall of defeat. Nothing I did was giving me what I wanted. I was leading in an organization, constantly over-doing and over-pleasing. I just couldn't say no, so I did more. As I did more, I became more exhausted, depleted, and resentful. I felt crushed, and I didn't not know what to do. I could see that I was over doing, but I didn't know how to stop. Was this the initiation into *un* becoming for me? I didn't know it at the time, but yes, it was.

I've studied as a spiritual leader, a psychologist, an educator/trainer, a public speaker, a brain nutritionist, a hypnotherapist, and a leadership coach for over thirty years. I've worked as a spiritual director for children and women, guiding and directing not only their spiritual lives, but their psychological and emotional lives. I also worked as a psychotherapist in a psychiatric hospital, helping deeply wounded youth and families find their way. Following that, I set up a private practice as a psychologist, providing one-on-one, group, and family counselling for more than 18 years. During that time, I also worked as a professional speaker, a workshop designer, and a facilitator for the corporate world (and I still do). Now, I offer leadership and brain coaching for individuals and organizations. But although I 'know' a lot, it has really been through my *personal* journey of *un* becoming that I learned the most important lessons.

I have been privileged to sit across from thousands of women in private, vulnerable, and deeply honest conversations. I have learned that they each experience this 'pushing'—in many different ways, but always as a way to try to find their value, the belief that they are enough. I researched, read, explored, and experimented with ways to help myself and my clients. Through this journey, I have discovered there are key principles that, when understood and then practiced, can create the life we all desire, can lead you to becoming you.

You are enough is a simple, yet profoundly transformative message when you work it into your life. When you believe deeply you are enough, you will no longer push against yourself, your life or others. This manual and workbook will assist you in unleashing the life you really desire. It will help you do your inner work, the work of discovering what you really value and want, who you really *are*, and then removing the barriers standing in your way so you can live the full, expansive life you long for—and live it with joy!

The boulder of *I'm not enough* is a heavy burden to bear, and you may be starting to realize that pushing this boulder is getting tiresome, and perhaps even exhausting.

What if you really believed that you mattered? That you are enough?

This book is designed for women who are ready to live in a *different way*, a courageous way.

This book is for women:

- **Who want a breakthrough in their life**, and know they are still pushing the same rock up the same hill and are tired of doing so.

- **Who have prayed, meditated, and read every self-help book available,** and who still find themselves discouraged like Sisyphus.

- **Who want transformation simplified,** where a few concepts can start a process of *un* becoming to become who you really are.

- **Who are ready to dive in.** For the women who want a deep sense of peace within and calmer minds and lives with less desire to be and do more.

- **Who need a little more direction** to focus on what is truly them.

Un **becoming is a path toward 'you'.** This book is for you if you are ready to *un* become the person you've been striving to be to instead focus on becoming *you*.

What does it mean to *un* **become?** The *un* becoming process outlined in this book is about unravelling what is not really you; the 'not enough' beliefs, the behaviours—like perfectionism and people pleasing and over achieving—that drive you to do more in order to 'be enough'. *Un* becoming this 'you', the 'you' that you've created in order to feel like you are enough, involves noticing, understanding, and then taking action. What you *un* become was not the real you in the first place. As I mention in the following pages, this process will be uncomfortable, because you will be giving up long-held beliefs and behaviours that, for some of you, may have become ingrained and has become your identity.

What could happen if you *un* become what you've created and become *you*? Would you feel less guilty, overwhelmed, and stressed? Would you pursue some of your dreams? Would your relationships be more enjoyable? Would there be more room for joy in your life? I know the answer to these questions: Yes!

What Is Different About This Book?

- **This is one book with many interrelated concepts.** This book is about many things: self-compassion, limiting beliefs, self-care, neuroscience, brain health, boundaries, building connections with others, spirituality and more. It is a book about how these elements relate and support each other.

- *Un* **becoming involves several aspects of your well-being.** It requires that we address our psychological, emotional, physical and spiritual well-being while understanding how each of these pieces are connected.

- **This book covers the 'how' of practical steps**. It's all here for you, with interactive questions and exercises to help you *un* become in order to become. We start with awareness, assessing yourself, and action for change.

- **These concepts work.** In this book, I present what I have discovered within my thirty-plus-year career as a psychologist, therapist, brain health coach, workshop designer and facilitator, professional speaker, leadership coach, spiritual leader, and researcher of personal development. I also draw on my multi-field education in psychology, leadership, adult education, hypnotherapy, and brain science. Everything in this book represents the exact same concepts that I teach in my workshops, retreats, and coaching sessions, and that I practice in my own life. I have experienced *un* becoming to become myself, and I have witnessed the lives of many women who have done this work with me.

- **There is simplicity in transformation.** My clients have taught me how applying these foundational concepts, sometimes only one or two concepts continues the flow of integration that generates personal transformation.

- **Changing is easier with support.** We all need the support of a community, or a guide with whom you can be real, vulnerable, and open as you discuss what is shifting on your journey.

- **Changing with the support of other women provides an important sense of community and greater growth.** I've designed this book such that you can work through it on your own, *or in circle with other women.* In fact, I recommend the latter. The guidelines for the group process are outlined in the Appendix.

The truth is that much of the information in this book has been available for a long time. Yet, so many women are still struggling with the same old story: over-doing, over-giving, withdrawing, self-criticizing, burning out, and remaining unfulfilled. This book will help you break that cycle by showing you how to stop *pushing* and start *becoming*.

You are enough. You do enough. Un becoming is the way to become who you really are. This is the transformation toward being enough.

This is the new way.
You are enough.

Becoming and *Un* Becoming

> *"We only have to become what we truly are."*
> —Oriah Mountain Dreamer

This is the new way to become you. You need to uncover and unravel what is not you. We need to *un* become.

Becoming You is a call to the journey of creating a whole, integrated inner-world so that your outer-world is the life you desire.

Let's begin.

Do you have your journal ready?

Take Your Time with These Introduction Questions and Exercises to Start Your Process

1. Who are you right now? What are you feeling and experiencing at this point in your life? Who are you being in the world right now?

2. Create a list of everything that you feel and do, but that you don't want to be feeling and doing. Write this out as a story or in a list.

3. Continue to express these thoughts as a poem. You can also draw, sketch, or doodle who you are right now.

4. Review what you wrote, doodled or sketched. Journal how it feels to see your life this way and how it felt to express it.

5. If you allowed the real 'you' to emerge and started to engage in a new way of believing and behaving, what could this do for you? What could happen if you got rid of what isn't 'you'? As you imagine what could happen, what does this feel like?

6. What would you like to be different in your personal or work life? What would you like to get out of your time spent in this workbook and on yourself?

7. Review what you wrote and express what you desire in a poem, drawing, sketch, or doodle.

8. Look at the two expressions—your life now and the way you want your life to be. What do you notice? What do you feel? Do you feel ready to fully commit to yourself?

   How can you be supportive of yourself as you take this journey of un-becoming? What might you need? What are you ready to do for yourself?

The *un* becoming that you will focus on in this section will help you move from where you are in the present to where you want to be. It's not a race, so take your time.

Section Two

Un Becoming—How?

Chapter One

Self-Compassion—Creating the Foundation for *Un* Becoming

Gently go within, inside, deeper, breathe, allow some space to rise.
Begin to notice all the many pieces of you.
The broken, shattered, and misshapen shards.
Those that are sharp and rough, some with bloody edges.

Those which don't seem to fit,

And want to shrink into the shadows....

Notice...

Breathe...

Allow space to rise...

Notice the smooth pieces, the soft ones, the lovely shaped ones,

The ones that reflect the light
and are lined with gold and sometimes hidden.

Notice...

Breathe...

Allow space to rise...
Embrace them...

All of them, the shattered and the smooth,

Allow them...

Breathe...

Hold them... .
With love and compassion.

I remember drawing how I felt about my life several years ago, when I was in graduate school. I drew scribbles of black and dark colors. I filled the page with how I felt on the inside. I was studying to be a psychologist, but more than anything, what I learned during that period is that no amount of academic information could make me happy. I was sad, and angry which made me get busy trying to fix myself. A constant sense of "push" was overwhelming, depressing, and exhausting me.

I wasn't sure how I was going to get through it, but somehow trusted, hoped, that I would. I didn't even know how I got there, but I knew that I'd been in that place for a very long time. I had just never paused long enough to acknowledge it. This time, I had to. I couldn't live my life the way I was.

Like Sisyphus, I was pushing and doing the same thing over and over and over again, hoping to get a different result. A few days later, I thought about what my life could be if I was peaceful, calm, loved, and completely okay with myself, if I believed that I was enough. An image slowly came into my mind's-eye of a large row of treasure chests spread out along a shoreline. I wondered what this represented, and I sensed that perhaps these were treasures which would help me become who I really am. I hoped so. I had no idea what was hidden within those chests, but I trusted that I would find out when I needed to. Looking back, I realize that I needed to uncover what was hiding beneath the surface of myself to see what was driving all my sadness and exhaustion. My head was filled with beliefs that I wasn't enough. As I journeyed along, a series of treasure chests opened, and that dream became my path. It guided me to find hidden gems to help me *un* become.

When we are driven by the messages that we get from society and ourselves, we are like Sisyphus—we focus on the boulder in front of us. We can see nothing else, so we keep pushing. But stop for a second, and ask: What if Sisyphus had begun to practice self-compassion? What would it have looked like?

Self-compassion provides comfort in discomfort, allowing us to love ourselves in the midst of pushing our boulders. Yet, self-compassion doesn't seem to come naturally to us. Instead, we self-judge, and we are critical. We continue to push, always against ourselves.

I imagine Sisyphus's inner dialogue would have sounded something like this:

I hate this f** boulder. It's huge, and it's all their fault that I am pushing it up this stinking hill. I didn't do anything that anyone else wouldn't have done. It's not that bad. I'm not that bad.

Sisyphus didn't look within. Instead, he externalizes all his problems. He blames. If he was to look inward with self-compassion, the conversation could be different. The conversation might even go like this:

I am only human. That doesn't mean that I'm perfect, but it does mean that I sometimes make mistakes. But I can't keep carrying that weight with me. If I ignore it, this boulder will likely get heavier. I am scared of facing who I am and what I have done. It is true, I am flawed. I have to try to be honest with myself and others about this. What if the boulder is my guilt? Maybe avoiding what I did was making this boulder larger than it needed to be, and maybe ignoring how I really feel made the boulder heavier. Yeah, this is tough, but I have to look at myself with some sort of love and acceptance, or I will just run. Run from it all. Or even worse... I'll. Just. Keep. Pushing.

Sisyphus certainly had time to reflect on himself. If he had taken that time to look within, he would've been forced to be honest about who he really was and what he had done. With time, and a little self-compassion, he perhaps could have taken responsibility for his actions instead of externalizing the blame. Blame is often what we do when we're not able to take an honest look at what is inside of us. We try to avoid pain by turning our gaze outward. You can only really work on 'you' with self-compassion. Otherwise, you will keep running from it all. Or. Just. Keep. Pushing.

Why did Sisyphus keep pushing? Maybe at some level, he believed that he deserved the punishment. But no matter what we've done, we always have an opportunity to look within and view ourselves with compassion. Only then can we begin the process of forgiving ourselves, which is the antidote to self-judgment.

Self-compassion means loving all of yourself, your dark and your light. It is paying attention to what may be beneath your surface and doing so with more self-love than self-judgment. It means seeing, feeling, and knowing everything about yourself, and then accepting the whole you. Self-compassion helps you see and love your whole self, your failures and successes. This is how we heal. This is how we become.

When we view ourselves and our frailties with contempt and self-judgment, we feel worse—this leads to avoidance. Compassion is how we help ourselves accept what is beneath the surface. What is beneath the surface has been put there because we are hurt and afraid. So we hide it. You are not alone if you find this difficult. Many of us do.

There are two important aspects of self-compassion to help you *un* become:

- Self-compassion involves being *with* your feelings rather than pushing them away. Be kind to yourself as you notice feelings during distressing situations.

- Self-compassion involves changing your self-imposed scripts, those negative judgments that overwhelm you when you believe that you have failed or when you experience a setback. We all have scripts like that: *That's stupid; I should know better; other leaders/mothers/friends don't act this way; how could I be so dumb? Why did I let that happen again?*

One of my leadership coaching clients, who has been navigating her way through self-compassion recently, shared her story with me:

> *At first, I resisted this notion of self-compassion. I couldn't see how being kinder to myself would help anything. I was so overwhelmed at the time, and I did not realize that it was my own voice in my head, telling me to do more, to do it better and to do it faster. People are watching, so don't screw it up. That was causing me to feel completely overwhelmed. I couldn't turn my mind off at night because I had to figure everything out for the next day, before I could come even close to relaxing, and it all had better be perfect. I knew I was a perfectionist, but I had no idea how to change it. The small steps I took to be kinder to myself, surprisingly, helped me a lot.*

This client says that she began to see her whole self, not just her *bad* self. She became a lot less anxious and much more resilient.

How did self-compassion work for her?

Before self-compassion, she didn't have a self-care practice. She wouldn't choose to think kind thoughts about herself. With self-compassion, she strengthened her mental resilience by focusing on what she had done well, not what she hadn't done (self-compassion). On her walk home from work, she would review what she did well that day, big or small, and through these seemingly small practices, she began to feel more joy. She was less in her head, she became more present, relaxed, and she smiled more. When negative thoughts about herself emerged, she would remind herself that *it's okay to feel anxious or worried,* and then she could reframe those thoughts. This felt better. She felt less anxious.

Before self-compassion, her brain was on overdrive, reviewing everything she did wrong. One day, after she had started practicing self-compassion, she told me about a positive work experience that would have normally sent her into a tailspin of negativity and anxiety: She was receiving criticisms from her boss about an important project. She was in a new leadership position and naturally wanted to do well, so receiving negative feedback from her boss wasn't easy. As the conversation unfolded, she was able to catch her thoughts going to self-judgment (e.g. *I'm a failure and I can't do anything right.)* and as a result, her breathing was rapid, and she started to feel anxious and overwhelmed. She noticed what was happening, so she paused, breathed, dropped her shoulders, and focused on staying present. She was able to say to herself: *that's okay...it's okay to feel nervous or even defensive right now.*

Over time, she was able to hear what her boss was actually saying instead of the negative story in her head. She became ready to hear that her performance needed improvement in one area. She didn't like the feedback, but she could hear it without cycling into shame (*I'm bad*) or blame (*they're wrong or they don't understand or this is their fault*). Her mind responded with fewer negative thoughts and she didn't become as overwhelmed with anxiety or fear. She could focus, hear, and understand, and then she could move forward with more ease.

For her, the practice of self-compassion also improved her confidence. Think about it: if you're constantly dwelling on negative things about yourself, how confident can you feel? For me, it was a beautiful experience to listen to her share about all of these changes: her face became softer, her voice was less pressured, and she looked me in the eyes, fully, without looking down or away. She smiled more, and her words were not chosen carefully—they just flowed from within her. She was becoming who she really is, and she was beginning to believe that she was enough.

How to Start Applying Self-Compassion

- Allow yourself to feel what you feel, without judgment. (We focus on this in Chapter 5, Emotions.) Catch your negative thinking, thoughts like *I shouldn't feel this way*, or *they didn't mean it*. Allow and accept those feelings. They are there for a reason.

- Reframe the situation. For example, tell yourself: *This is just feedback. It does not mean that I am a bad person.*

- Create an 'I am' mantra for yourself. It could be something like, "*I am loved*", "*I am whole*", "*I am enough*". Say this to yourself often. Say this first thing in the morning, throughout the day, and again as you fall asleep at night.

- Journal your experiences. Be aware and write down the feelings that come up when you are being hard on yourself. What self-judgmental thoughts emerge? What feelings show up as a result of these judgments? Write down the feelings and practice accepting them. Remember, what you feel is okay and necessary.

Self-Compassion Summary: What We've Seen So Far

- You can respond to your thoughts with more gentleness and kindness. Speak to yourself in a supportive manner. Any perceived failure you may have is not really 'you'.

- You can notice your judgmental thoughts and flip the script to *I am enough*.

- Remember to honour how you feel. Be with your feelings without judgment.

Self-Compassion Exercise: Checking In

1. **Write a letter of affirmation to yourself**. Include your talents, your gifts, and your positive characteristics. What is the true, unique you? Write in the third person if you like (for example, *Susan is a person who is always there for others. She is kind and thoughtful.*).

2. **As you write this letter of affirmation and review it notice and record:**

   - What was this process like? Comfortable? Uncomfortable? Awkward?

   - What did you feel as you wrote this letter about you? What emotions emerged?

   - Notice your thoughts. What were you saying to yourself? (For example: *this isn't true, this sounds arrogant, this is bragging, others don't see me this way, I hate focusing on myself*, etc.) Write it down. Allow and accept your thoughts. They will tell you a lot about your beliefs about yourself.

- Was there anything you learned about yourself, thought of differently, or noticed in a deeper way?

- Did this exercise help you connect with more self-compassion?

Self-Compassion is a life pattern aiming to change your thoughts to a more positive direction, and always in a gentle way. Over time, your choices and behaviour will be more in line with your desires. You will become motivated to live your life from a place of love, and not fear. Anxiety is often the result of believing you are not enough. What if some of your anxiety was due to the story you tell yourself about yourself? For the client I mentioned earlier, her anxiety and low confidence was in large part due to her own self talk. Self-compassion will shift you out of self-destructive thoughts and create a landing for you, a safe place to live from.

As you work through the rest of the book, each chapter will continue to draw from self-compassion. I encourage you to continue practicing this mindset of love toward yourself.

The Power of Self-Care to Help You Become More Self-Compassionate

In my group coaching sessions, we work through the same concepts outlined in this book. We start by committing to three self-care practices a day to create and preserve the belief of being enough. This sounds simple, and it is. It's also effective. In fact, the most effective practices of self-care are those practices which take only a few moments per day. Regular and consistent practice can create powerful change.

My clients report that self-care on a regular basis helps them feel more confident as they set boundaries and let go of responsibilities other than their own. Self-care is helping them *un become*.

Within a recent group, I had the pleasure of witnessing shifts in several women by our second meeting. In just two sessions, they were softer, calmer, more centered, and kinder to themselves.

They had begun to treat themselves as if they had value. One woman shared her self-care practice of taking just fifteen minutes at the end of each day to sit quietly and reflect on what was good about her day. Another shared how she had more courage and less guilt when she politely declined a request of her time. Another was beginning to focus a little more on physical exercise. Their new attention to themselves was creating an important shift toward being enough. This is what self-care does.

Shifts from *I am not enough* to *I am enough* lay the foundation for learning other healthy and *un* becoming oriented behaviours. You can find a list of self-care practices in the Appendix.

Reflection: Self-Compassion

Choose one or two of the following questions for reflection.

1. Self-compassion involves being with your feelings without judgment.

    a. How are you doing with this presently?

    b. Can you think of a recent time where you weren't kind to yourself? What *could* you say to yourself that would show yourself more compassion?

    c. How does that moment feel to you now?

2. Self-compassion involves changing the script from judgment to acceptance.

    a. How do good are you at doing this, currently?

b. Can you think of a recent time where you could have changed your script? For example, instead of *why did I just do that?* (which implies that you should know better), could you have said, *I am doing my best*. In your example, what could you say to yourself to be self-compassionate?

c. As you say it to yourself now, how do you feel?

3. How might you incorporate self-compassion into your daily life? Finish the sentence: 'I can be more self compassionate by ....'

Learning to Just *Be*

settle in the here and now
reach down into the center
where the world is not spinning
and drink in this holy peace
feel relief flood into every cell
nothing to do
nothing to be
but what you are already
nothing to receive
but what flows effortlessly from the mystery into form.
nothing to run from
or run toward
just this breath
awareness knowing itself as embodiment
just this breath
awareness waking up to truth.

—Danna Faulds

Allow yourself a few moments to slow down and breathe. Read this poem slowly and allow the words and feelings they evoke in you to gently deepen. Move into your center. Be here. Be still. Breathe.

Remember, self-compassion is the foundational 'way' in which you start to create the *I am enough belief.* This foundation is essential for the next steps as you begin to *un* become who you created yourself to be.

Take your time exploring and practicing self-compassion before moving onto the next Section.

You are enough.

Chapter Two

Limiting Beliefs Part I
What Are Limiting Beliefs?

*". . . if we allow ourselves to be shattered by these experiences,
they can have a transformative impact on us: they can lead us to
become appreciative participants in mystery, instead of controllers."*
—*Jerome Miller*

If you believe you are enough, you will feel calm much of the time.
You won't feel driven to be more and do more.

If you believe that you are *not* enough, you might think that you
need to be perfect. You might think that you need to please others or
overachieve to have value, love, and respect. If you believe that you
are not enough, you will likely feel anxious, nervous, or sad—maybe
not all of the time, but some of the time. If you believe any of one
of these, you may say yes when you want to say no. You may drive
yourself to over do.

What Is a Limiting Belief?

Limiting beliefs are those perceptions and false assumptions we have about ourselves which are simply not true and limit us.

These beliefs sometimes go unnoticed by us. Because we have lived with them for so long, they have become so unconscious to us that we think they *are* us.

The awareness of feelings, even subtle ones, is part of your *un* becoming. When you are unhappy (even if it's beneath the surface) and don't notice, you will engage in behaviours to try and make yourself feel better. You may try to be perfect, to please people, or over-achieve to feel better about yourself and make the unhappiness go away. This behaviour will end up reinforcing the belief that you are not enough because you never get enough-ness by doing.

As women, we usually *desire* connection and *fear* rejection and abandonment. A set of limiting beliefs—or false perceptions of ourselves—often arise to fulfill what we want and what we avoid. Limiting beliefs lead us to do things we don't want to do, and as we do, we move further away from our true path and our true selves. Unravelling our limiting beliefs and the choices we make because of them is a crucial part of *un* becoming. It's where we start.

By uncovering our limiting beliefs and then challenging them, we regain the power to choose the life we want. This begins to lead us out of situations where we are holding ourselves hostage by the expectations of others and our own unrealistic expectations. We can begin to choose rather than be controlled. This moves us from the world of *shoulds* to the world of *choice* which moves us to the *freedom* to be who we really are.

Practicing self-compassion is also necessary to this process because as you begin to see yourself and the limiting beliefs that are driving you more clearly, you will feel uncomfortable. *Becoming you* means embracing all sides of you, including your dark ones. It's not about fixing you.

Embracing is a loving act, and love heals. Take your time and be gentle with yourself as you move through the information and exercises in the pages ahead. Consider how you can practice self-compassion as you become more aware of your limiting beliefs. For example, try to repeat *I am enough* as you begin to realize why you do what you do.

Your limiting beliefs may overlap and intersect. Identifying, noticing, and paying attention to them is part of the process of transformation and *un*becoming. If you don't notice your boulder of limiting beliefs or understand how you may have created it, it could not only fall backwards, but crush you. Noticing and doing something about your limiting beliefs will transform and empower you.

- **Your behaviour starts with your beliefs**. Many people focus on behaviour and try to change at that level, with little success. If you recognize and uncover the limiting belief that is driving the behaviour, your success will be sustainable.

- **Limiting beliefs make your boulder larger.** They increase the size of the hurdles you face, and they drive you to do the things that you don't want to do. With these beliefs, you make choices to try to be enough, but these choices and resulting behaviours make you feel worse, not better.

- **Limiting beliefs punish us.** They make us feel like we are lacking, and they push us to fill the hole of *not enough*. That hole is like a bottomless pit, and the more you try to fill this pit, the worse you feel about yourself.

- **Limiting beliefs are often hidden from us.** Just like Sisyphus working in the underworld, our limiting beliefs hide beneath the surface of our consciousness. This doesn't lessen their impact—it increases it. Some limiting beliefs remain dormant or hidden for years or decades, and we don't see the ways they are affecting our lives. This may be one of the reasons we don't change. We actually don't even realize that a boulder is there! Or we know that there is something more beneath the surface, but we are too afraid to go there, or we don't know how. I have noticed this with many of my clients, and it usually takes a lot of self-compassion and self kindness to see what we don't want to see. It's hard, and it takes time.

- **As an introduction to this concept,** the diagram below illustrates how feelings follow thought.

- **Many of us are more aware of our behaviour than our beliefs.** We recognize our drive to try to make everything perfect by over-planning or over-doing, or our tendency to not say *no* when we know we need to, but we are less likely to be aware of the *beliefs* driving our behaviour.

Beliefs lead to emotions that lead to behaviours that reinforce beliefs. Thinking, feeling, and doing reinforce each other in a cycle.

As you review the diagram following, reflect on your own life, the way you feel, your behaviours and perhaps what thinking (beliefs) might be driving these.

Exercise: Write out what might be true of you, in each of these areas: Thinking, Feeling/Emotions, Behaviours.

Unhealthy Belief Cycle

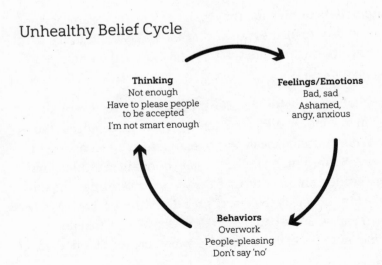

Thinking
Not enough
Have to please people
to be accepted
I'm not smart enough

Feelings/Emotions
Bad, sad
Ashamed,
angy, anxious

Behaviors
Overwork
People-pleasing
Don't say 'no'

Understanding Your Limiting Beliefs: Examples of Three Primary Types

There are lots of limiting beliefs, but I am focusing on the three I believe have the greatest impact on women. They are:

Perfectionism—the need to do things right or perfectly, most or all of the time. Perfectionists undertake a relentless pursuit of doing more, doing it faster, and doing it perfectly. Perfectionism is the belief that our human value is found in how well we do things.

People-pleasing—the fear of disappointing others, or the need to please in order to feel valuable and worthy. People-pleasers see their human value as being directly tied to how other people view them, and how well they are liked.

Over-achieving—the need to succeed, to be the best, to be the top of your game all the time and to surpass others at all costs. This belief, like the others, is driven by the need to feel valued, and it feeds our own sense of self-respect.

Let's take a closer look at how these limiting beliefs might be playing out in your life.

Limiting Belief Exercise

To help identify the limiting beliefs which may be creating challenges for you, please complete the exercise below.

Rate each statement 0—4:

0 = I never experience this
1 = I rarely experience this
2 = I sometimes experience this
3 = I often experience this
4 = I experience this a lot or most of the time

Section A

☐ I always *have to* do things right, or I always have to do my best.

☐ What I do never quite measures up to my own expectations.

☐ I tend to procrastinate as a way to avoid not doing things imperfectly.

☐ I feel defensive when others point out my mistakes or errors.

☐ I think that others may think less of me if I don't do things perfectly.

☐ I feel bad about myself when I don't get it right.

☐ I feel like I should try to do everything 100% right, 100% of the time.

☐ I get stressed or tense when things aren't just the way they should be.

Section B

- ☐ I tend to take criticism very personally.
- ☐ I feel guilty when I say "no" to people who ask for my help.
- ☐ I feel pulled to help many people.
- ☐ I believe that the approval of others is important.
- ☐ I feel upset if others are disappointed in me or angry at me.
- ☐ I always go the extra mile to help other people.
- ☐ I find it hard to say no to others in need.
- ☐ I feel guilty a lot when I say no to others.

Section C

- ☐ Success in life is very important to me.
- ☐ I often feel that I could do better or achieve more.
- ☐ I feel like I always need to be productive or busy.
- ☐ I sometimes feel inferior to, or jealous of, those who are more successful.
- ☐ I feel better about myself when I am successful.
- ☐ Failure is not an option for me.
- ☐ I tend to believe that those who succeed, who have fame, outstanding careers, etc. are happier than people who are not particularly successful.
- ☐ I tend to feel nervous or guilty if I'm not working hard, producing, or moving forward.

Scoring:

Add up your scores for each area and record here.

0 = not at all
1 = rarely
2 = sometimes
3 = often
4 = most of the time

Section A—Your Perfectionism total: _____
Section B—Your People-Pleasing total: _____
Section C—Your Over-Achieving total: _____

Results for each area:

- **8 or less = Little to no issue in this area**. Perhaps this is an area you've been addressing for some time, and you are experiencing positive results. If that is the case, congratulations on your hard work! It is also possible that you are not aware of how this belief is impacting your life, so keep an eye out for signs of this issue in the future.

- **9–16 = Moderate challenges in this area**. You may struggle from time to time with this belief, and it gets in the way of your decisions, time management, and boundaries. You may be aware of how this is impacting your life.

- **17–24 = Moderate to high challenges in this area.** This may be an area of concern for you. You are likely getting pulled into believing that you need to behave in a certain way in order to have value. It may be difficult for you to slow down, to take time for yourself, to relax, to be assertive in a respectful manner, to or set boundaries. You may feel angry when you receive criticism or feedback, and you may become defensive or withdraw.

- **25—32 = Significant challenges in this area.** You may find it very difficult to say "no," to set boundaries with others or even on your own high expectations, to be assertive, to let go, to slow down and/or to relax. You may feel resentful because of all the demands on you. You may become controlling of others as a way to get what you want. You may drive yourself to over-do or achieve. You may even consider that being a martyr in this way is a badge of honor. It may be time to address this issue in a more intentional manner.

Reflection Questions and Exercises

1. Write down the area above (i.e. perfectionism, people-pleasing, or over-achieving) that you struggle with the most and why you think this is happening for you. Take your time.

2. What might you be trying to overcome in your life with this limiting belief? (e.g. a feeling of being less-than, not enough, or inferior).

3. How do you think this limiting belief is impacting your life at work and at home (e.g. your ability to set healthy boundaries for yourself, your stress level, your relationships, your time management, your choices, your emotional, mental, and physical wellness, etc.?)

It is helpful to understand how limiting beliefs create patterns of perfectionism, people-pleasing, and over-achieving. We are trying to avoid the feelings that come from not believing our value, and we compensate. We believe that if we *do more, please more, achieve more*, and *do it better*, we will feel better about ourselves. This behaviour distracts us, and we may never create the time or space to notice what is happening within. It's as if we learned a long time ago that in order to feel safe, loved, valued, and respected we needed to become something we are not.

What if Sysiphus had recognized his limiting beliefs and how they were getting in his way? To recognize this, he would have had to stop pushing and give himself space to acknowledge how tired and frustrated he was. Then, he could have considered what he was trying to accomplish with all of this boulder-pushing. Like Sisyphus, many women know the things they do, but they don't know *why*. Many know they over-do, over-give, and try to do everything perfectly, but the *why* is not conscious. Limiting beliefs are often the reason.

Summary: Checking In

Unless we unravel our limiting beliefs, we will never become who we really are. We will remain trapped. If your limiting belief was a mountain, then you might be going *around* it instead of *through* it. Continually going around the mountain will always bring you back to the same place. Avoidance is usually due to fear, and a lack of awareness contributes to this. Facing our limiting beliefs involves going through the mountain. The way you have been addressing this up to now is going to change. What got you here will not get you there.

Sisyphus never faced his boulder. He kept doing the same thing the same way, over and over again, getting the same results. He couldn't see what he couldn't see. The boulder was his entire focus, and this prevented him from looking deeper and actually seeing what the boulder was all about.

Here is what we have learned about limiting beliefs:

- Limiting beliefs hold you back from becoming who you really are.

- There are three main limiting beliefs: perfectionism, people-pleasing, and over-achieving

- Awareness of limiting beliefs is a critical step to *un* becoming, for it allows you to see what is at the root of your distress and unhealthy behaviours.

- Always consider how self-compassion can support you as you go beneath the surface to understand why you do what you do, and the limiting belief behind this.

In the next section, we will spend more time talking about each limiting belief and how they can affect our lives. But for now, let's focus on what we can do about them.

Questions and Exercises for Review and Reflection:

Choose one question below and reflect:

1. When have you shown self-compassion toward yourself in the last while? What was it like to be more kind toward yourself? How did it feel?

2. How might self-compassion help you be more okay with your current entanglement with perfectionism, people-pleasing, and/ or over-achieving?

3. Review your "I am" self-mantra. How are you continuing to repeat this to yourself as you are becoming more aware of how your limiting beliefs are affecting you?

Take it deeper:

4. Review again which limiting belief tends to show up for you the most.

5. Finish the sentence: "Learning more about my own limiting beliefs may help me to.................."

Self-compassion exercise—The Letter:

1. Contact two people that you trust deeply. Perhaps choose one person related to your professional world and one person who knows you more personally.

2. Ask the individuals to describe your positive characteristics, how you show up for them, what you mean to them, and the way they see the value you bring to the world.

3. Ask them to send their response to you in writing.

4. Once you receive these letters, read them over slowly with an open heart. Let yourself feel what you feel which might be a mix of emotions. You might feel encouraged, grateful, happy, or uncomfortable. Notice what thoughts emerge, for example: *are they really telling the truth?* Or maybe: *they're just saying this because I asked them to. This isn't really true.* Notice if it's uncomfortable or awkward to allow their words to sink in. Try to stay as open hearted to their truths about you as you can.

5. Write down your feelings and thoughts that result.

Once you have this information, choose three key positive things that were said about you, for example: thoughtful, humorous, passionate. Reflect on these observations from time to time, perhaps when you go to bed or first thing in the morning. Allow the truth of these positive statements to sink in. Practice saying these three descriptors of yourself over and over again.

Say it in this way: "*I am kind.*" "*I am loving.*" "*I am smart.*" Breathe deeply as you meditate on your strengths and your gifts. Consider incorporating them into your "I am" self-mantra.

Going Forward: I encourage you to continue practicing daily self-care and reflect on one or all the questions below. And remember: You can find more self-care suggestions in the Appendix.

As you engage in self-care:

1. Take notice how this attention to yourself is changing how you feel, how you view yourself and if it is beginning to reflect in your decision-making?

2. What is decreasing?

3. What is increasing?

Uncovering what we believe about ourselves can be uncomfortable, perhaps even frightening. Notice if you are experiencing a desire to avoid this work. It's okay. We all hide, and we all avoid. We start and we stop. I notice this discomfort in a lot of the women I work with. You are not alone. And please keep trying. This work helps you know what you need to unravel, and it is an important step in *un* becoming.

You are enough.

Chapter Three

Limiting Beliefs Part II
Understanding the Impact
of These Beliefs

"The unexamined life is not worth living."
—Plato

Now, more than ever, we need to learn how to let go, slow down, and create balance in our lives. So many of us are racing to do more, to be better, to prove ourselves, to achieve our dreams, and to change the world. We are doing more than ever, and some of us turn success into a sign of how important we are. It is easy for us to *do* as a way of avoiding the mountain in front of us. Doing because we believe we are not enough may make us feel like we are making headway, but it actually creates another trip around the mountain.

Reflection: As you move through this chapter, consider what you learned about your limiting beliefs in the last chapter. Which belief is limiting you the most right now?

Limiting beliefs are relentless. Our mind becomes attuned to anything external that we believe will give us more or less value. For example, if we notice someone else getting the accolades we want, our brain goes into high alert and triggers our fear of not being enough, which can start a spiral of fear and anxiety.

Limiting beliefs drive busyness, and they are a distraction from feeling. Many of us would rather stay busy than experience sadness, anger, grief, or hurt. But as long as we distract ourselves with busyness, we can avoid the clutter, noise, and negative thoughts in our mind. Continuing to avoid diminishes our well being.

In this section, we will be spending more time diving into each limiting belief. Pay close attention to each of them. You may find that one of the limiting beliefs where you scored lower in the exercise is actually more present in your life than you thought. You may also recognize some of the other ways that a particular limiting belief is affecting your life. Be open. This is to help you *un* become.

Perfectionism

The need to be perfect makes us think, *I am not enough unless I behave perfectly and do things perfectly.* It says, *If I am perfect, I have value.* But we never get there. Perfectionism can be tricky because we can always be or do better—so how do you know if you're engaged in a healthy pursuit of expansion, or if the need to be perfect is controlling you? Perfectionism also impedes our sense of freedom and sense of calm. We can't go to bed because we need to do just one more thing, or when we make a mistake, we can't let it go. We might not even be able to sleep. We keep thinking about what could've been done or said better.

Perfectionism at Work

Someone who believes that they need to be perfect may become hurt and act defensive when receiving feedback about their less-than perfect project or performance. They can be overly hard on themselves, and they may be hard on others as well. They may work long hours and may never be happy with their results (or anyone else's). They may expect even more and are rarely satisfied. Perfectionists are often hurried and impatient. Sometimes, they withhold ideas because they don't want to risk getting it wrong. They might talk a lot as a way to prove their worth by showing how smart they are or to prove what they are doing is right. Perfection shows up in unrealistic deadlines and over-promising. The result of perfectionism at work and in life is a loss of trust in yourself and others; from that place, asking for help seems like an impossibility, and this feeds the cycle of believing that you can only rely on yourself.

Perfectionism is a complicated belief because it's a big lie intertwined with experiences of empty success and short-lived happiness. Perfectionists may succeed, but they are not satisfied. Perfectionism doesn't make us feel better about ourselves—it makes us feel worse because when we *do* fail, and we will, we are devastated. Some of us pick ourselves up, try harder, and engage in an endless cycle of pushing. Remember Sisyphus? Some may become so exhausted from this push toward perfectionism that we eventually give up and withdraw.

What a Perfectionist Does

A perfectionist, despite personal achievements, will downgrade their successes, their physical appearance, and so on. They sometimes take daily inventory of how they've done, but they never measure up. For example, with feedback, performance evaluations, and reviews, the perfectionist will hear the negative and bypass the positive. It's like the negative comments have a megaphone and the positive comments are barely audible. Some perfectionists may over-inflate their achievements, or they may lie to cover up the pieces they don't want known.

Perfectionism Beneath the Surface

Because perfectionism is the pursuit of being enough, we can never get there. At some point, we will experience frustration and become discouraged. The underlying driver is fear, but it might be deeply buried.

A Story of Perfectionism

I remember a young woman who attended one of my workshops. We were discussing the ways that we put pressure on ourselves and how this can hold us back or drain the enjoyment out of our tasks. She was a superb craftswoman, and her husband and others affirmed it. She wanted to express herself through her work, but she was plagued by nagging thoughts that she wasn't good enough. To overcome these nagging beliefs, she tried to do her work perfectly. When she started her creations, she was often paralyzed and sometimes couldn't even complete them. Even though others loved her work, she didn't believe them, so she pushed herself to keep going. It was excruciating for her. Her fear of being a failure, of not doing a perfect job and having someone notice it was just too much. Eventually, she compounded guilt about not being able to complete anything, and her perfectionism stopped her from enjoying her gifts.

Perfectionism shows up differently for all of us. It might show up in your professional life, where the need to be perfect paralyzes you. Or you may work long hours to do everything perfectly, then get irritated and annoyed by anything less than perfect. It may show up in your personal life, where you want the perfect meal, family gathering, birthday, or holiday celebration. You may be holding yourself back, never able to enjoy your gifts and talents because of your need to be perfect. Perfectionism can create anxiety and overwhelm.

Reflect on and Review Perfectionism

1. Do you think you have any tendencies toward perfectionism? If so, in what areas of your life are you trying to be perfect?

2. How might perfectionism be impacting you? Irritation, being overwhelmed, withdrawing, resentment toward others, doing too much, being overly responsible?

People-Pleasing

People-pleasing is one of the most deceptive limiting beliefs. We believe that we are doing good, being kind, and helping others by pleasing people. In reality we are doing this to control the way other people see us—by trying not to disappoint and by giving others what they want. The people-pleaser, above all else, wants to be liked. They believe that this is what gives them value.

People-pleasing looks good—it is praised and reinforced

People-pleasers often hear things like, "*You're so nice!*" or "*We love you so much!*" This reinforces the cycle. We keep pleasing to be liked and when we are liked, we believe that it gives us value. We wear ourselves out in the process and often put ourselves last.

What People-Pleasing Does

The people-pleaser may cause a lot of problems—not just for her, but for her family, her other relationships, and for those she leads and works with. If she is a leader, her attempt to not disappoint might prevent her from making tough decisions. Her need to be liked is greater than her commitment to do the right thing. Communication may not be clear. She may defer hard decisions to others. She may become dishonest or minimize issues in an attempt to cover up perceived mistakes or failures. Trust becomes eroded. The focus ends up being on her and her need to have people like her, instead of what is best for the organization.

Similarly, people-pleasing causes problems in our personal lives. It may make us override our own needs out of a fear of disappointing others. We end up living in a world of *shoulds*, with no real choices. We feel constant guilt for not measuring up, doing enough, or being nice enough.

Remember: the motivation behind people-pleasing is not to please others. It is self-serving. It is an attempt to control others' view, so we are liked and can avoid the fear or anxiety that arises when people are disappointed in us. People-pleasing is never about them. It is always about you.

People-Pleasing has the Opposite of the Intended Effect

People-pleasing results in the opposite of what we think. We are not respected because at some level, people see us as dishonest, or even weak. Even our friends, colleagues, or loved ones can't quite put their finger on why they feel this way. People may become frustrated with us because of our indecision, our lack of boundaries, or our over-apologizing.

People-Pleasing Beneath the Surface

Women who engage in people-pleasing are often quite angry and resentful beneath the surface, especially if this pattern has been there for a while. When we don't get back from others at the same level that we're giving, we become angry. As women, we tend to shove down what we need and side-line ourselves for so long that we become very angry. Accessing and admitting this anger means confronting our people-pleasing beliefs: we feel that we must be kind and nice at all costs. Many women who engage in people-pleasing are not even aware of the anger that lives beneath the surface.

Reflect on and Review People Pleasing

1. Now that you know more about people-pleasing, think again. Do you have any tendencies toward people-pleasing? If so, what areas of your life might you be people-pleasing as a way to ensure people like you?

2. How might people-pleasing be impacting you? Irritation, feeling overwhelmed, withdrawing, anxiety, resentment toward others, doing too much, being overly responsible... Is there anything else?

Over-Achieving

Over-achieving is the drive to do more, to be the best, to achieve success in order to feel valued, respected, and loved. It is often our need to be seen, cherished, respected, or adored for our achievements. This brings on yet another never-ending push which can drive women to undermine and attack each other instead of supporting each another. Another person's success seems to be a direct threat to the over-achiever.

But wait! Isn't it *good* to want to achieve or do better? Yes, of course it is. But it can be problematic when we can't stop, can't slow down, or when we run over others who get in the way of our success. Some of us may push ourselves into relentless driving, such that we stop choosing. The drive is to feel valued and loved, which will never be filled by even the greatest successes.

Overachieving Professionally

The over-achiever is constantly looking for recognition. She may aspire to get more education, more training, more certificates, and more awards than others. These ambitions may get in the way of her own health and wellness, as well as her creative pursuits or any number of ways of being which might not seem purposeful enough.

Workaholics may fall into this category. Workaholics derive so much self-worth from their work that they can't stop. They have to do more and be more in order to believe that they have value.

Because they don't believe they are enough, over achievers try to gain value through their successes. Once again, this is fear. Fear of not being enough or doing enough. Fear of missing out. Another feeling which may lurk just beneath the surface is jealousy. Jealousy of others' achievements can trigger the limiting belief of not doing enough or not moving ahead fast enough.

Impact on Others

If you are an over-achiever, people may respect, you but they may not really *know* you. Therefore, you may not really connect emotionally with others. There is a distance. Over-achievers often talk a lot about their work, their next big idea, and their latest achievements or successes. They want to be respected for what they do, so this is their focus. They may have difficulty talking about other things with friends and family, thereby affecting these relationships. When they do talk about personal things, it's often about how well they are doing. They do not want to be viewed as a failure, so they hide their failures from others and are not vulnerable. They may get bored easily if life isn't exciting or they're not after the next "big thing." Because the focus is often on the over-achiever, friends and family may not feel important.

Over-achieving beneath the surface

Over-achievers may not take time for personal pursuits or self-care or relaxation because they are driven for more. They may have difficulty slowing down, relaxing, doing nothing, or taking time for themselves. This pattern is not sustainable and over time, the over-achievers may become completely exhausted, or simply burnt out.

Reflect on and Review Over-Achievement

1. After reading this chapter, do you think that you have any tendencies toward over-achieving? If so, where do you see over-achievement showing up in your life?

2. How might over-achievement be impacting you? Do you feel tired, overwhelmed, anxious? How is this affecting your time for yourself or your health? How is it affecting your close relationships?

Limiting Belief Exercise: Pros and Cons

Now that you've reviewed the concepts of perfectionism, people-pleasing and over-achievement, let's move on to a more focused exercise to help you recognize more deeply how your limiting belief(s) is affecting you and your life, and how it is getting in the way of you becoming the real *you*.

I invite you to complete an exercise to help you recognize the impact of one of your limiting beliefs. You will explore the pros and cons of each belief. To start with, consider one of the three main limiting beliefs: perfectionism, people pleasing, or over-achieving.

What is a Pro and What is Con?

Pros are what your limiting beliefs give you, even when they cost you. Sometimes people have difficulty coming up with the pros, because the reasons for this particular behaviour may be hidden from you, but we don't choose and repeat behaviours that don't give us something. Pros are what you are trying to gain from this limiting belief. You can bring your pros to the surface by deeply reflecting on *why* you do what you do.

The pros are also what you will be giving up when you stop acting on this limiting belief. For example, as you give up people-pleasing—which gives you a sense of being liked—you may have more conflict with people because you start being more assertive, or because you stop saying "*yes*" every time someone asks you for a favour. People may become uncomfortable with the "new you." You may be giving up a false sense of ease in your relationships. You may have to face disappointing people and all the discomfort that come with it.

It's important to take a close look at the pros, because they are what hook us and allow us to buy into the limiting belief in the first place.

Cons may be easier to recognize. The cons are the reality of what you experience when you act on your limiting belief. Ask yourself, *what are the problems that arise because I hold this belief?* Think about your stress level, the quality of your relationships, the quality of your alone time, the quality of your health and wellness, and the quality of your thoughts. Are they critical or kind and accepting? The quality of your recreation time and the quality of your relationship with your career are also relevant here.

Take a moment to read the following example and then complete the exercise below.

Example of Pros and Cons Exercise

Limiting Belief: Perfectionism

Limiting Belief Statement: "I need to do things perfectly and be perfect to feel valued."

Pros:	Cons:
How does this belief give you what you want?	How does this belief create difficulties in your life?
Pros:	Cons:
• I will be viewed as a great friend/Mother/leader/employee • I will do things perfectly and receive great satisfaction from this • I am extra responsible • I may get rewarded at work • People can always count on me to do things perfectly • I don't let others done	• I am stressed from trying to do things perfectly • I do a poor job of taking care of my own needs because I work long hours • I am not honest with myself or others • I become angry at others easily for their lack of perfection • My relationships are not honest • I am overwhelmed • I am resentful • Stress and unhappiness increase • I rarely ask for help. • I have to do it all.

Now You Try:

Write out the following. Refer to the example above for ideas and assistance.

The limiting belief I want to address: _____

My limiting belief statement: _____

Pros: Why you do this? What you gain from acting on this limiting belief?	**Cons:** How does this limiting belief contribute to difficulties in your life? How does it affect your choices, your relationships, your work, your self-care, your stress, and your ability to set boundaries? Be specific. With whom and in what circumstances?

Reflection

Now that you've completed this exercise and understand more deeply why you engage in these limiting beliefs, you can have a better sense of their impact. Can you see that you engage with these beliefs to feel valued? Can you also see how limiting beliefs actually *diminish* your sense of value, your belief that *you are enough*?

When you lay out the pros and cons like this, it makes it easier to see. We engage in behaviors related to our limiting beliefs because we *think* that they will bring us more love, more approval, more praise. But in reality, they erect barriers between us and our loved ones, they reinforce our fears, and they make us put our own needs on the back burner. They reinforce our feeling that we are *not enough*.

Pain in *Un* becoming

Accept and expect pain as you become aware of your behaviors related to trying to be perfect, to people-please, or to over-achieve. You might feel frustrated right now because you see more clearly, the harm your choices have done to you or you are unsure of how to change your patterns, or maybe you are frustrated because you find yourself still struggling with this. Breaking longstanding habits is difficult, and sometimes it feels like regret or loss. This is part of your journey.

Rest assured, the remainder of this book will help you move forward to *un* become so you can continue becoming *you*.

Summary

- Know that awareness is power. Awareness of your limiting belief gives you the power to act on the limitations that hold you back.

- Living with limiting beliefs and the behaviours that follow can cause a lot of pain for you. Remember, some choices can feel good in the moment, but they are only a short-term fix.

- Be mindful of being self-compassionate as you become aware of your limiting beliefs and their impact on your life. Use your "I am" mantra when you start to feel down or discouraged while reflecting on limiting beliefs.

Going Forward

Keep up with your daily self-care activities. Take time for you. This is an important act of self-compassion and a way to hold space for yourself as you see and heal beneath the surface.

The good news is, that becoming more aware of your limiting beliefs gives you power to *un* become, and this is part of the path to becoming *you*. These limiting beliefs are false, and they are not part of the real you. As you have taken the time to reflect more deeply on the beliefs that drive your behaviour choices, take a moment to be gentle with yourself. Say a few words of kindness in a calm, slow manner. You are courageous.

This is hard work. Breathe. Be kind, and remember:

You are enough.

Chapter Four

Limiting Beliefs Part III
Breaking the Addiction
and *Un* Becoming

"The most terrifying thing is to accept oneself completely. Your visions will become clear only when you can look into your own heart. Who looks outside, dreams; who looks inside, awakes."
—Carl Jung

The Emotional Impact of Being Addicted to Our Limiting Beliefs

What would happen if we realized that what is actually holding us back is not our inability to do more, to do it better, or to make people happy, but rather the belief that our value hangs on these things? What would happen if we were able to let go of those beliefs?

Unfortunately, letting go is not so easy. If limiting beliefs gain traction in our life, they can empty us. Limiting beliefs can have us behaving like addicts. I meet plenty of people who think they can just stop pleasing or striving for perfection, only to fall back into the same old patterns. They then beat themselves up for their failure to change, feel worse and engage in the behaviors again in order to avoid the pain.

There is that boulder again. Remember: the behaviours change when we change our beliefs and the beliefs change as we change our behaviors.

Addictions hook us emotionally, and so do our limiting beliefs.

They make us feel enslaved to our fears. Our attempts to stop these behaviours can cause intense anxiety because we are simply trying to meet deeply-rooted needs. As you unravel these beliefs and change your behaviour, you will likely feel intense discomfort. You might even feel desperate and begin to seek new ways to feel valued.

When this happens, return to self-compassion (accepting what you feel with acceptance and kindness), as it is the only way through. It might feel scary, especially in the beginning, but have faith and keep moving forward.

Addictions mix our motives.

We say we want to kick our habit, but do we really? When we are kicking a habit or shifting a long-engrained pattern, we tend to feel pulled in opposing directions. On the one hand, we want to over-achieve, be perfect, or over-please because in the short term, it gives us something we long for: value. It is our attempt to think we 'are enough'. On the other hand, we know the behaviour has negative consequences, so we want to stop. Then we feel guilty about not stopping, and this makes us feel worse. It's as if the boulder goes up the hill and comes back down in the same breath.

Addictions impede our freedom.

An addict feels little to no choice in the matter. If we are hooked on a behaviour, we will do anything to justify it. We will lie to ourselves. We will say *it's not that bad*, or say things like, *after all, I'm just helping this person out*, or *I'm working late just one more time because I have a stellar work ethic.* When our freedom to choose is impeded by our limiting belief, we do not choose what is healthy for us. We are driven in one direction, and this, in itself, has eliminated the possibility of a genuine choice.

Letting go of behaviours driven by our limiting beliefs will be uncomfortable.

When we get an award, a promotion, or praise for our good deeds, our brain releases chemicals that make us feel good. When we are addicted to these chemicals and repeat behaviours in order to get our hit, we deprive ourselves of choice.

When we choose to say *"no"* to a request that does not fit us or our values, or when we say *"no"* to the relentless pursuit of doing anything perfectly, we will feel the pain and absence of the chemical satisfaction we are accustomed to. This is real.

Your brain won't like it at first. You may feel worse before you feel better. The discomfort is showing us that we are experiencing withdrawal symptoms, but it is in shifting the behaviour that we start to break the addiction. This difficult decision and the change you implement puts you on the path to *un* becoming.

Questions for Reflection—Part I

Choose one or more questions to reflect on:

1. How might your limiting beliefs (perfectionism, people-pleasing, and/or over-achievement) hook you emotionally? How might you feel *addicted* to them (e.g. you feel hooked, they impede your freedom, they mix your motives)?

2. How are your limiting beliefs mixing your motives? Where do you want to stop doing what you're doing, but feel like you can't?

3. How might your limiting beliefs be impeding your freedom to be who you really are?

Now that you've taken some time to reflect on your limiting beliefs and their impact on your life, I invite you to consider how to *diminish* the impact of these beliefs. Think about the limiting belief which holds you back as you move through the rest of this chapter.

Suggestions and Questions for Reflection—Part II

Read the following and decide on one or two things you want to start working on for the next while and you then journal your reflections as you consider a specific situation. Think about a difficult or challenging situation or relationship. Work through a few of these steps below with this challenge in mind:

1. What is the limiting belief that is showing up and how could you challenge this belief by asking: *what would you say differently to yourself in this situation?*

2. How might you remind yourself that you are doing your best, that you are okay, and that you don't need to be perfect or please others?

3. How could you adjust your personal expectations? If you are less hard on yourself, what could you let go of?

4. How will you manage and be prepared for the guilt as you begin to step back? Feel the guilt. Accept the emotion coming with it. It's part of the process.

5. Who can support you? Talk to other women, friends, co-workers, or your spouse about where you find yourself stepping-up and where you might be struggling. Learn to ask for help when you need it.

6. How can you practice self-compassion during this process? What can you say to yourself? Breathe. Be kind to yourself. Speak kindly to yourself.

Continue to Journal: With this challenge in mind, ask yourself: what could you do differently? How would that feel? How might beginning to unravel these limiting beliefs in your life, help you become who you really are?

Being Honest with Yourself

One of my recent workshop participants scored herself "low" on the same limiting beliefs assessment that you completed earlier. She did not see herself in any of these beliefs, so she thought that she didn't have an issue. As we moved into smaller groups, she began to reflect on some of her choices. She shared about how busy she was outside of work, how over-extended she was, how confusing this seemed because she enjoyed all the activities and responsibilities she took on (e.g. mixing motives). She seemed to be in conflict: was this really a choice for her, or was she being pulled to please? On one hand, she knew that service to others is important to her and that she enjoyed it, but on the other hand, she was feeling tired and overwhelmed. I asked her to consider if any of these volunteer activities were getting in the way of her health and wellbeing, or her time to pursue other activities or dreams. As she re-evaluated, the limiting belief which showed up was over-achieving. She began to recognize that she was addicted to over doing, pushing herself more and more. She began to notice how she was making the people she helped and those she worked with, more important than herself. She just felt the need to keep pushing and doing more and more.

As she became more honest with herself and the group, she shared, that she was not only feeling tired, but she was often the one who picked up the slack for others. She hadn't allowed herself to feel the anger and resentment beneath the surface until now. She had pushed these feelings down, judging them as bad, and judging herself for having these thoughts. The more she didn't admit how she really felt, the more she continued to over-extend herself. She began to realize that over doing, was keeping her from noticing herself, taking care of herself.

In short, she kept pushing the boulder.

This participant needed to ask herself how she could serve others *and* be healthy and happy. Limiting beliefs lock us into one thing— our need to please, be perfect, or over-achieve. Limiting beliefs don't allow us to be annoyed at others *and* be a good person.

Questions for Reflection—Part III

The following questions help you determine if you are perfecting, people-pleasing or over-achieving. Consider using these questions not just now but going forward as your guide to determining if you are out of balance.

1. **Are you perfecting? People-pleasing? Over-achieving?** Think about a situation or challenge that you are presently involved with, or something that is coming up in the near future. To determine if you are approaching this with balance (consideration for yourself and the other) or not, consider the following questions:

   - Is this commitment negatively affecting or limiting your finances in any way? How so?

   - Is this commitment negatively affecting or limiting your mental health? Your emotional health? Your physical health? How so?

   - Is this commitment limiting you and/or those you love in any other way? Is this commitment limiting the pursuit of your own goals or dreams? How so?

   - Is this commitment limiting you or those you love in any other way that has not been discussed? How so?

Coming to Grips with Your Addiction

You may be thinking your life is pretty good and maybe it has been pretty good. Yet, many of us may relate to the following excerpt from *Velvet Elvis,* by Rob Bell, more than we'd like to admit:

> *In one moment of enlightenment, my therapist and my wife were helping me drag up specific events from when I was in my early teens. I was remembering them like they were yesterday. I remember the encounter, what was said, what I did, how I reacted and what it did to me. Now, I come from a family where I was loved and supported and yet I have junk from way*

back then. What we discovered is that some of these experiences produced a drive in me to succeed and prove myself and show others. Sound familiar? Part of my crash came from my failure to identify these forces until recently. I have been pushing myself and going and going and going and achieving and not even really knowing why. It is easier to keep going than to stop and begin diving into the root causes. Some people don't know how to stop. They are driven and are achieving and are exhausted and don't know how to say they're tired. They are scared to look weak... I think that's why so many of us push ourselves so hard. As long as I'm going and going and going, I don't have to stop and face my own pain. Stopping is just so difficult.

This certainly sounds familiar to me. Some of you may not have experienced severe trauma in childhood or growing up, yet many struggle with being kind, loving and accepting toward themselves. We seek acceptance and a feeling of *enough-ness* to survive. Any form of neglect causes harm. Your past may have been traumatic, or your past may have been similar to Rob Bell's. Either way, we often grow up with some sort of lack, and we grasp and push to have our needs met by external sources, instead of looking inward to fill the hole.

The Healthy Belief Cycle

As we unravel the power of limiting beliefs in our life, we start to create new, healthier ones. We start to believe that we are enough, and we start to become who we truly are. When we believe that we have value, positive feelings begin to emerge, and they turn into healthier behaviours. Remember, feelings follow thought and behaviours follow feelings. As we change the behaviours that are driven by limiting beliefs, we create more space for ourselves. Our confidence grows, our trust grows, and we become stronger. We will actually become kinder to others.

Recognizing and unravelling your limiting beliefs (that we all have) is *un* becoming and it is in this process that we also start to become who we really are.

Exercise: Consider what you desire in each area—beliefs, emotions, behaviours—and after reflecting on this diagram, take a few moments to write out your thoughts.

Beliefs lead to Emotions that lead to Behaviours that reinforce Beliefs.

Healthy Belief Cycle

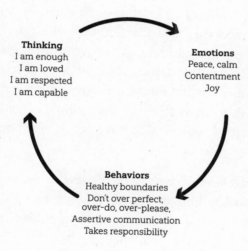

Thinking
I am enough
I am loved
I am respected
I am capable

Emotions
Peace, calm
Contentment
Joy

Behaviors
Healthy boundaries
Don't over perfect,
over-do, over-please,
Assertive communication
Takes responsibility

The process of *un* becoming to become you, feels bad sometimes.

This process of noticing how our limiting beliefs drive us to feel and behave in ways that are harmful to us, can be hard. This awareness is the first step and is key to change. The pursuit of transformational change, from *un* becoming the person you strove to be for so many years to *become* the person you really are takes courage. It is actually a good thing when the shadow feelings and beliefs emerge. It means that you are changing. These uncomfortable feelings mean you are *un* becoming. So hang in there.

Sisyphus never stopped to reflect on the boulder or why he was pushing it. For an eternity, he lived in the underworld the same way he lived on earth. We too may eternally push when we allow ourselves to be controlled by our limiting beliefs. In recognizing that we have them, why we engage in them, and how they impact us and others, we can start to let go of our boulders. We can start to change. With awareness, we can start to live a new way. Limiting beliefs are what keep you from becoming you.

It is uncomfortable and sometimes scary to look beneath the surface and see our deeper beliefs and feelings, but when we look, with kindness and acceptance, we might just find the richest parts of ourselves. Compare our lives to a garden: we know healthy plants don't just grow on the surface—they require roots to grow deep into the soil to access water and nutrients. For you to grow stronger and healthier, you're also going to need to reach deep down. Then, you can love those deeper parts of yourself that have not received nourishment for a long time. Maybe never.

Remember, awareness of what you believe is power. Continue to notice when you are hooked into a limiting belief like perfectionism, people pleasing or over-achieving. Then pause. Tell yourself the truth: *I am enough*. Know that this all takes practice and time. In fact, this will be practiced over and over throughout your life.

Visualization Exercise to Release Addictive Limiting Beliefs

Take your time and set aside about twenty minutes to do this exercise. Repeat it anytime you feel you need to.

1. Think of a situation or relationship that is challenging for you, that causes you some distress. You may want to start with a low-grade distressing situation and move your way up to something more painful.

2. Write down two or three of your false beliefs about yourself based on this situation. (For example: *I don't matter. I'm not good enough. I must be perfect. I can't disappoint others. They don't like me. They don't think that I can do this.*) It may take some time and patience for you to recognize what you are saying to yourself.

3. Write down the truth beside each false belief. (For example: *I matter. I am a great worker. I am enough. I do enough.*) Focus on just one truth that resonates for you and circle, highlight or underline that one truth. Think about that truth for a moment.

4. Close your eyes and take a few deep breaths. Allow your mind to clear, and as you focus on breathing, count *3... 2... 1...* very slowly in your mind. Allow yourself to relax. Repeat this a few times.

5. Next, visualize the distressing situation. Imagine you are there. What do you see, hear, feel, and smell? Notice the surroundings. What do they look like? What color are the walls? Notice the sounds. Is there a fan blowing? Are there any subtle background noises? Notice what you are sitting on, standing on. What does it feel like? Who else is there? What are they saying or doing? This visualization is meant to take you into that time in your mind.

6. Next, as you hold this memory, begin to say the one truth to yourself. Repeat it very slowly, at least three times. (For example: *I matter.*) Notice how you start to feel relaxed.

7. Notice what you feel when you really believe this. You may feel calm, peaceful, or confident when you really believe what you are telling yourself. Notice where you feel this in your body. Try to maintain the feeling for at least 12 seconds. You can do this by imagining that you are breathing that feeling into every part of your being and body.

8. Continue to be aware of your breathing.

9. Repeat Steps 4 through 8, as necessary.

10. Open your eyes when you feel ready. You will intuitively know when.

11. Review and Journal: Write out your experience of this exercise.

Note: Isn't it amazing, how telling yourself the truth makes you feel better? It can be a relief to finally see this and face this.

Limiting Beliefs Review

We have learned a lot about limiting beliefs. Let's take some time to review.

Reflect on at least one of the next three questions:

1. As you near the end of this chapter, what are some of the ways you can begin to unravel the behaviours coming from your limiting belief(s)?

2. What can you say to yourself when you find yourself in a pattern of perfectionism, people-pleasing or over-achieving to help unhook you and lessen any self-criticism?

3. Is there anything you are ready to let go of (beliefs or behaviors) related to perfectionism, people pleasing, or over-achieving? How might you begin to do that?

4. Is there anything different you could or could not do?

Going Forward

Self-care enhances self-compassion. Self-care and self-compassion provide the safe landing from which to let go of limiting beliefs. What can you do for yourself that brings a deeper sense of well being into your life? Consider practicing 'one' thing daily. Just for you.

Here are a few suggestions (there's more self-care ideas in the Appendix):

- Write in a gratitude journal.

- Review all that went well today.

- Set a positive, affirming intention at the start of your day, such as joy, peace, calm, or focus.

- Read a few pages from an inspirational book.

- Daydream.

- Connect with nature.

By shifting your attention to yourself with daily practices, you will continue to shift to a deeper knowing of being enough.

You are enough.

Chapter Five

Emotions Allow Your *Un* Becoming

"If you don't go within, you go without."
—Zen Proverb

Sink deeply into the swirl of the ocean

*It is here within the depths
That you will find yourself.*

Your Shadow and your Light.

Finding Your Inner Peace

To *un* become, we need to acknowledge, accept, and allow our emotions. *Un* becoming is not just learning an emotional process. It also involves releasing emotions that are stuck, ignored, and hidden. This can be hard work. Emotions are a part of us, and we need to feel them in order to heal. If we ignore, we don't explore.

Un becoming is not about pushing, just ask Sisyphus! It is about allowing, and the same applies when we're talking about our emotional life. We can let our emotions guide us to something deeper, and we do this by allowing them to be there. To feel them. To discover what they are telling us. And then to heal.

This process may rattle you at times. It may make you believe that your boulder is falling backwards. But this is important: it's in the falling that we notice what really matters.

The process of allowing our emotions helps us understand what is going on beneath the surface. By accessing how we feel with self-compassion, we can unearth a limiting belief, discover a value that we are clinging to, or put our finger on something else that may be causing the distress. When we uncover an emotion, we also uncover the reason for it, and our practice of self-compassion gives us the courageous space to feel it and go deeper and then determine what we need.

Take your time as you read through these symptoms of inner peace and reflect on your own life.

Symptoms of Inner Peace by Saskia Davis

- A tendency to think and act spontaneously rather than acting on fears attached to past experiences.

- An unmistakable ability to enjoy the moment.

- A loss of interest in judging other people.

- A loss of interest in judging self.

- A loss of interest in interpreting the actions of others.

- An inability to worry (this is a very serious symptom!)

- Frequent overwhelming episodes of appreciation.

- Frequent acts of smiling.

- An increasing tendency to let things happen rather than to make them happen.

- An increased susceptibility to the love extended by others as well as the uncontrollable urge to extend it.

As we *un* become to become who we really are, these symptoms occur with increasing frequency.

Questions for Reflection

Choose one to two questions for reflection and journal your thoughts:

1. As you review the above list, consider the items that you want to experience.

2. How might self-compassion assist you in feeling more peace? Take your time with this one. This could be big.

3. Consider your primary limiting belief: how has recognizing and accepting this belief, and sharing this information with others (if you have), brought you a level of peace? Why might that be?

4. Given what you've read on emotions so far, how might attending to your emotions and learning how to honor them help you feel more calm and peaceful?

The Value of Emotions

As you read this chapter and reflect, I invite you to give yourself space, to feel more.

Emotions don't have much value in our culture

Many people are afraid of them, or they don't understand what to do with them. One of my colleagues told me that she views emotions negatively, something that needs to be fixed. Some say that there is no room in the workplace for emotions. What do you think?

In my experience, we can choose to ignore, deflect, or run from our emotions, but diving in is the way to *un* become.

Emotions have immense value in our lives

They allow us to love deeply, feel passionately, and feel rage or anger at injustices. Noticing and acknowledging our feelings helps to protect us against our own and other's boundary violations. Not only that, the exploration of emotions is one of the most valuable and insightful self-care practices that we can engage in. When we explore our emotions, we uncover deeper understanding, deeper awareness, and thereby deeper healing. We allow for release, healing, and growth to occur. And we can then choose differently, create different action, based on the 'noticing' of what we really feel.

Negative emotions help us recognize one of four things:

1. A boundary is being pushed, challenged, or stepped over, either by someone else, yourself, or a situation.

2. A limiting belief or the sense of not being enough is being triggered.

3. A combination of the above: we've been violated, we're engaging in critical self-talk, and we're beginning to believe that this was our fault, that we failed, or caused it, etc.

4. Something difficult, such as a personal loss, has happened and you are experiencing grief and/or other emotions.

Even though there are thousands of self-help books and business books that address emotional intelligence, too many of us remain grossly unskilled at identifying and dealing with our emotions. Why do you think that is? We get stuck on the fact that admitting how we feel can make us vulnerable or that feeling various emotions means we are weak, not perfect or not doing enough, for example.

In her book *Women's Bodies, Women's Wisdom*, **Dr. Christiane Northrup,** says that our emotional patterns become biology. "If we don't work through self-destructive thoughts and subsequent feelings, our destructive thoughts and suppressed emotions set ourselves up for physical distress because of the biochemical effect that emotions have on our immune and endocrine systems."

When we understand this, breaking out of emotional patterns takes on a new level of significance.

Case study: Understanding Your Emotions

An entrepreneur and professional woman was struggling within her family. She was over-doing, over-giving, and she did not ask for help. She planned family trips, booked the tickets and hotels, planned family gatherings and meals, and cleaned up after every event. She was always the contact person. Her family were all in, and they allowed her to over-do. She did not realize it at first. From her perspective, she expected her family to know what she needed, so she never told them. For years. Perhaps she didn't realize that her need to control the planning and execution of these events was part of her perfectionism and that not asking for help and over-doing was because of her over inflated need to please.

Through all of those years, she didn't allow herself to feel the growing resentment deep inside her. She was so driven by the need to please in order to feel valued, and her need to control things to be perfect that she just kept pushing her feelings down, all the while telling herself to just *let it go. It was fine, no big deal. I love my family.* She believed that she shouldn't feel overwhelmed or resentful because everything she was doing was for her family and they weren't bad people (*they would never take advantage of me*), so she continued to push herself past her own limits. She told herself to suck it up, so she stuffed her annoyance and resentment inside. The real challenge was not with them, but with herself. She over-gave because she did not want to be viewed as unkind. She had been the giver, the organizer, the planner, and the doer for her family members for a very long time. She took control of everything so it would be perfect. Both of these, being the perfect family planner and being the one who pleased everyone had become part of her identity. She believed her over-pleasing gave her value although she was not aware of this until she began to do the work. Her perfectionism which showed up as planning everything (control) kept her anxiety down, temporarily. To unravel this, and *un* become, she began to face that her need to please her family was actually for her, not them. She then started to notice and take responsibility for how she was feeling.

Changing meant some tough, courageous work. She started following the emotional processing steps I outline in this chapter. It was hard to admit to her anger and resentment., She viewed it as "mean" until she reframed it with self-compassion and called it *being human* instead. She slowly and gently began to allow herself to feel frustrated and overwhelmed. From here, she could see that her perfectionism and people-pleasing had been causing the problems. She began to acknowledge, accept, allow, and process why she behaved this way.

It all started with accepting and allowing how she felt, without judgment. With self-compassion.

As she acknowledged and accepted her feelings, she could be more objective about what was creating these feelings. This gave her space to reflect on *her* actions and she started to think about how she could do things differently. Prior to family gatherings, she started asking others to take a turn with food prep and clean-up. She started to do less. She began asking others to do more when planning family trips. She engaged in self-care on a regular basis, journaling in the morning, and reading something inspiring daily. She found this allowed her to be more courageous and gradually set more boundaries. As she began to let go of over-giving to others, she had more time to give to herself. She's become a stronger person who is clearer about her own needs and more decisive. These changes have helped her believe more deeply that *she is enough. This* situation, and her time of reflection on herself and her behaviors, helped wake her up. To herself. To her emotions. To her needs.

Questions for Reflection

Choose one to reflect on and journal your thoughts:

1. Journal your thoughts about this story. What relates to you?

2. What are you tolerating right now, and not fully feeling as a result?

3. How could the process of acknowledging, accepting, and allowing your feelings make a difference to you?

Following the Thread of Feeling

I adamantly believe that the only way to release emotions is to face them. Whether you stuff them deep down or lash out, these are both ways of avoiding the responsibility of your emotions. How many times do we jump to a solution without truly understanding the problem? Without following what I call *the thread of a feeling*, you may apply a solution to the wrong problem. You can't make a good decision without knowing how you truly feel. Our tendency is to gloss over feelings and not fully acknowledge them.

Let me share a story about how the thread of feeling can bring deeper insight.

Case study: Thread of Feeling

A bright, young woman named Alice came for leadership coaching at the recommendation of her organization. When we started our first conversation, she shared the organization's view about her: they thought that she had immense leadership potential and that she could move up the corporate ladder as a result. However, she did not appear to be too interested in this prospect, yet on the other hand, believing it was wrong to think this. She felt confused and pressured. We talked about this in more detail.

"Confusing because?" I asked.

"Because I don't want this, but it seems like I should."

"Pressured because?" I asked.

"It's just too much. It feels overwhelming."

So, as we followed the threads of how she *felt* rather than what she *thought*, we were able to get to the bottom of the issue. She felt confused and pressured because a higher position was an achievement, but it meant less time for herself. She had seen other burned out and stressed out leaders. She didn't want that for herself.

"What should be the first step in your coaching?" I asked.

"To figure out what my plan is. If it's not to move up the ladder, then what?"

I then added that it might be useful for her to determine what her values are, and she agreed.

It turns out she valued: work life balance, time with family, and the opportunity to lead and develop leadership skills.

When she identified her values, she gained the clarity to understand why she'd been feeling so much pressure. If she moved up the corporate ladder, it would impede time for a family and work-life balance. What felt right to her was to stay in her present position. This gave her time to develop leadership skills without additional pressure, and it also gave her time to focus on herself, her wellness, and her family. She needed this. She had been ignoring herself for a very long time at the expense of pushing herself.

How did we know it was the right solution? Because she felt relieved once she removed her self-imposed pressure to move up. She looked and felt more relaxed, signaling that this direction was congruent with her values.

It Is Not True that Time Heals All Wounds

That's like saying you can leave all the clutter and garbage in your cupboards and over time, if you ignore it, it will all just magically disappear. It won't. In fact, it will grow, and eventually rot. Emotions are the same way. Some feelings are like magnets that will build to a point where you may have no choice but to pay attention to them. They increase not decrease if you ignore them. Ignoring what you feel is ignoring yourself.

It is hard sometimes to let go of what is good
so that you can have what is better.

In my client's case, promotions seemed good even the right choice, but they would have cost her what she really wanted. Did she get through this quickly? No. As she released her expectation (which was really a 'should'—*I should move up the ladder. If I really am a skilled leader, I should go further*), she felt both guilty and relieved at the same time. She continued to struggle with perfectionism, which made her question herself. Doubts crept in from time to time as well.

Am I doing the right thing?

Shouldn't I be doing more?

Should I be pushing harder?

At these times, she worked on acknowledging, accepting and allowing what she was feeling. She determined that her feelings arose because of the pressure she put on herself. She decided that she would review her values to confirm and validate her decision. It was an easy, yet difficult decision to not climb the corporate ladder at this time. She didn't rule out the possibility of seeking a promotion at a later date, and she continued developing her leadership skills in her present position. Since she chose what was right for her, she created the internal space to work more deeply on herself. She worked on self-care and self-compassion, and she created new habits and practices to deepen her confidence and sense of calm. This gave her more clarity and energy. She worked on being less of a perfectionist because she knew that if she moved to a higher position, that belief and habit could overwhelm her. She embraced the *un* becoming process and as she did, the power she had been giving away to others *(The only right way is to be promoted and move up the corporate ladder.)* lessened and her trust in herself deepened. She didn't *have* to do this just because others' thought it was right for her. Letting that expectation go, created peace for her.

Questions for Reflection

1. What stands out to you about this story? Have you every felt conflicted like this?

2. How might ignoring your emotions now lead to more pressure later?

3. How might recognizing how you feel help you understand what you truly need?

Responding to Your Emotions: The Process

The following is a process you can follow when you are feeling troubled or are faced with something distressing.

Read this process over first, and you will then complete an exercise on your own. Take your time while you review this.

1. Acknowledge, Allow, Accept the Emotion:

    • Name the emotion if you can.

    • Locate where you feel the emotion in your body.

    • Stay with the emotion.

    • Be present with it and be patient with it.
      Remember self-compassion.

2. Ask why the emotion is there. Be willing to explore.

3. Explore what you might need.

4. Take appropriate action.

Now, we will work through this process one step at a time.

The First Step of the Process: Acknowledge, Allow, Accept the Emotion.

Try not to judge or criticize yourself for why and how you are feeling the way you do. Beliefs like these may emerge:

This is stupid. I shouldn't feel this way. They didn't mean it. This isn't that big of a deal. If I was really together, I wouldn't feel this way. Anger is bad. I feel guilty for having these thoughts.

If that happens, simply be aware. These thoughts may be subtle at first. As you begin to notice your judgmental and self-critical thoughts, you will begin to be aware of them. Feel what you are feeling. Name it. Notice and write down what you feel. Be patient and be kind, and just notice. Self-compassion.

Try not to be critical of yourself for having these thoughts. You might think that you shouldn't be judging yourself, that you should know better, etc. This is a sign that it's time to practice patience and self-compassion.

Feeling your emotions means that you are taking responsibility for them.

This is challenging because of three behaviors which can get in our way:

- We **blame**, which looks like putting our focus on the person or situation that caused the problem.

- We **shame**, which looks like putting the focus on ourselves and telling ourselves that we are somehow bad.

- We do **both**.

Allow yourself to feel the emotion, by trying to name it and then by focusing on where your body is holding it. For those who have difficulty naming their emotion, there's a list at the end of this Chapter. Understand that, for many women, naming emotions is difficult.

Our tendency to want to quickly find a solution to our emotions. Over-thinking shoves the feeling down deeper and keeps it in a never-ending cycle of activation. Our need to analyze the emotion is our attempt to control it and make it go away. This won't work because emotions don't want to be fixed. They want to be noticed.

Remember, you don't need fixing. You need to feel because feeling is part of how you value yourself.

Noticing what you feel is a bit like talking to yourself. As you are allowing yourself to feel and telling yourself that it is ok, and even necessary. Self-compassion is so important here, and having a kind, patient attitude toward yourself will help you hold the space you need to feel any pain which may surface.

Remember: Acknowledge, Accept, and Allow the feeling.

Let's consider a specific scenario to understand how the first step in this process works.

Feel the emotion. Acknowledge. Allow. Accept. Let's say you are upset at a co-worker for talking over you, interrupting you, and not allowing you an opportunity to finish your sentences.

You recognize that she talks a lot more than you do. You notice that you are feeling annoyed, but you ignore it by telling yourself that your co-worker is a good person, that she's just trying to do her job, that she doesn't mean it. You begin to argue with yourself. On one hand you are annoyed, and on the other hand you think that you shouldn't be because she's a good person. You also start to wonder if you should say something, and that brings up fear about a confrontation, so you try to talk yourself out of feeling annoyed. You don't want to have the conversation, so you ignore what you are feeling.

Do you notice the subtle lie here? If you allow yourself to feel annoyed at this co-worker, you tell yourself you are judgmental, which pulls you to continue ignoring the emotions you are feeling.

In the process illustrated above, you can be both annoyed *and* believe that your co-worker is a good person. This process allows you to feel the annoyance, to let the feeling be there, and to see where it takes you. You may feel it in your chest, and as you feel it, start to notice some anger. Emotions will intensify as you Acknowledge, Accept, and Allow. This is a good thing. They intensify because you are paying attention to them. Noticing.

You might need to talk yourself through it: *It's okay to feel this. There's a reason I feel this way. I'm okay. I'm human.*

As you allow this, your chest will start to relax, and you will breathe more easily. The emotion will likely diminish a bit.

When you have a way of allowing yourself to be with your emotion, you can learn how to address your emotions and manage how to express them in a way which is not harmful to others or yourself. It takes courage. *Fully* acknowledge, allow and accept your feeling(s) before moving on to the next step. Do this step *without* thinking about what to do. That will come later. If we think about that now, we will become afraid and have the potential to not fully feel what we need to.

The Second Step of the Process: Explore the 'Why' of the Emotion

Once you have allowed yourself to feel the emotion and accept it, you can move on to exploring what it is all about. This is what many refer to as *processing*. It doesn't mean that what happened is okay, but it means that what you feel is real. A lot of people's first response is to lash out or withdraw. Both of these reactions are signs that you are triggered. Be careful not to use *why* in a judgmental way. It is meant to help you understand what is going on, not to say, "*Why do I always do this?*" or "*Why can't I get past this?*" That kind of thinking is like saying, "*It's so stupid that I feel this way.*" This is judgmental.

Ask: *What is this about? Why am I feeling this? What happened to affect me this way?*

Ask: *Has a boundary been crossed? Have I allowed something in my life to cause this feeling? Did someone say or do something to make me feel this way?*

Ask: *Am I triggered by perfectionism, people-pleasing or over-achieving? Am I interpreting this situation to mean I am not enough?*

Once you determine the why of your emotion, write it down.

Reframe your feelings. Once you understand why you feel the way you do, you may need to reframe it. If your feeling arises because of unnecessary expectations on yourself, reframe it.

Repeat: *I am enough. I did enough.*

If your feeling arises because someone did something disrespectful to you, reframe any self-criticism you may have.

Repeat: *Even though I was treated this way, I am a good person, I do have value, and I am enough.*

If you received negative feedback about something you did that hurt someone else, allow yourself to feel this, and then reframe if necessary:

Repeat: *What I did was hurtful, and I am still a good person. I can change this behaviour.*

Reframing is powerful. Reframing trains your brain to believe in the good in you, and this can bring some balance to the emotion.

Validate your feelings

Using the example above, you realize that you are annoyed and angry because your co-worker talks over you, interrupts you, and does not let you finish talking. Validate your experience and your feelings. It makes sense that this annoys you. You are not allowed to express your opinions. Validating keeps your *why* objective without emphasizing or minimizing it.

The Third Step of the Process: Explore What You Need

Once you have determined what you feel, the reason you feel it and why, it's time to ask yourself what you need. Explore this and be honest. You may need to step back. You may need to do less. You may need to have a conversation to clarify what you need or want before you move forward.

Do you need to step back from someone or something? Do you need to have a conversation with someone?

As you consider the action, check in with yourself to see how you feel. If it is the correct action and one that is right for you, your emotions will align with it. You will feel peaceful, calm, or relieved. If it is the correct action for you, your physical body will also respond with alignment. Your chest will become less tight. Your stomach will soften and relax. You may, however, feel some nervousness about the action needed. That's okay and normal.

Continuing the same example, you realize that you really need the interrupting and talking over you to stop. How do you do this? You have a conversation. As you consider how you would feel if this behaviour stopped, you realize this is what is needed. When you consider doing nothing, you continue to feel stressed or overwhelmed or hurt.

The Final Step of the Process: Take Action

Take action. Have the conversation. We'll come back to this in chapter eight when we talk about courageous conversations. For now, set the boundary and step back. You may need to set a boundary with yourself. (We'll learn more about boundaries in Chapter Six and Seven.) Do what you need to do. Once you do this, review what you did. How did it go? How did it feel to set this boundary, create this change? Be self-compassionate as you review. You don't have to get this perfect.

In the co-worker example we have been walking through, you would plan for and have the conversation, pointing out the behaviour, the impact it has on you, and what you need from your co-worker going forward.

Practice Exercise—The Process

Think of a recent challenging situation. Go through the four emotional processing steps described above and write out your responses for each step. I encourage you to take your time, be patient and kind with yourself, and to practice self-compassion.

Summary:

1. Acknowledge, Allow, Accept the Emotion.

2. Ask yourself why the emotion is there.

3. Be willing to explore what you might need.

4. Then plan and take appropriate action.

Two Response-Styles to a Triggering Event: Over-React and Under-React

There are generally two responses to a triggering event: an **over-reaction or under-reaction.** When we **over-react,** we lash out, show anger, sarcasm, defensiveness, or attack. When we **under-react,** we pull away, retreat, withdraw, or ignore, Both are ways to manage our belief of *not being enough*. It's a form of protection. What is your typical style?

As we learn to be aware of our style, we can allow ourselves time to pause and go through the Four Step Process, starting with how you feel without judgement.

Questions for Reflection: Complete the Sentence:

1. I tend to over-react or become defensive when ....

   What limiting belief do you think is being triggered?

2. I tend to under-react, pull away, avoid, withdraw, or ignore when .,................

   What limiting belief is being triggered?

Emotional Self-Awareness: Feeling Words

To acknowledge what we feel, we need to have the right vocabulary. Some people simply say they feel *good, fine,* or *bad*. While those descriptors likely get close to the truth, they don't get at the heart of the feeling. They just aren't specific enough. Here is an example of a common conversation to illustrate the challenge in identifying what we feel.

Me: "So, when _____ happened, how did you feel?"

Client: "I felt disrespected." (The client usually goes on to share the details about what happened. They often tell me the details of the story rather than how it impacted them and how they felt.)

Me: "How did it feel when you were disrespected?"

Client: "I didn't like it."

Me: "What does that feel like to you?"

Client: (Pause) "I don't know. Not good."

Me: Pause....I say nothing. I am allowing them space to experience what *not good* feels like.

Me: "Hurt?"

Client: "No, not hurt." (Pause) "Angry. I felt angry."

Me: I begin to notice them feel the anger as they allow it. When they are ready, we can explore the why of this feeling.

This illustrates our human pattern, our difficulty in really knowing and naming what we feel.

What do you notice in this conversation? What might happen next for them now that they are able to name the feeling as anger and not disrespect? Disrespect is not a feeling. It is an action. By not naming the feeling, we are unable to access it, connect to it, honor it, or, in time, hold space it and move through it. It's important to find a way to name the real feeling.

I often invite my clients to refer to a fuller list, like the following, to help them determine what they are truly feeling.

The list is divided into four broad categories (mad, sad, glad, bad), with several more specific emotions below them. These categories were created by my colleague, Dr. June Donaldson, author of the bestselling book *Emotional SMARTS®*.

Review the list below. Know that as you review this list, the words will start to settle in your mind, and you will be able to access them more easily when you need to express your feelings You can refer to this list anytime.

Mad:	Sad:	Glad:	Bad:
Angry	Hurt	Happy	Lonely
Resentful	Hopeless	Content	Defeated
Frustrated	Helpless	Excited	Weary
Exasperated	Empty	Joyful	Overwhelmed
Rageful	Depressed	Elated	Anxious
Hatred	Miserable	Relaxed	Fearful
Annoyed	Defeated	Peaceful	Worried
Irritated	Discontent	Calm	Shocked
Impatient	Apathetic	Optimistic	Disgusted
Ticked off	Dejected	Satisfied	Depressed
Bitter	Upset	Loved	
	Grieving	Pleased	

As you go forward, reflect regularly on what you are feeling instead of what you are thinking. Practice being with yourself in this manner. You can practice this with any emotion, whether it is positive or negative. Remember that noticing where you feel the feeling in your body, helps you notice the feeling. Then it is sometimes easier to name it. Notice how much more comfortable you are becoming with knowing what you feel and allowing yourself to feel it.

Emotions—Summary

- Emotions are important. Like a lighthouse, they shine a light where a boundary may have been violated, and they can help you discover the deeper meaning behind the emotion.

- The Process to Working with Emptions is as follows:

  - Acknowledging, accepting, and allowing your emotions is an essential practice to unraveling what isn't you. This is self-care. This is self-compassion.

  - Next, you review the "why" behind this response.

  - Then, you explore what you need.

  - Then, you decide on the action.

- Practice will help you to become more comfortable with your emotions.

Questions and Exercise

Choose one or two questions to reflect on and journal your insights.:

1. *I presently handle my negative emotions by*..

2. *How does the way I handle my emotions help or hurt me and/ or others?*

3. *I struggle with accepting my emotions because*...............

Check-in:

1. How are you doing?

2. What is going well? What are you most proud of?

3. What do you need to do more of? Less of?

Choose one question to complete

1. **Self-Care**: Journal about the self-care practices that have been most beneficial to you and any changes you are noticing as a result.

2. **Self-Compassion:** Journal about your practices of self-compassion and what you are noticing.

3. **How does self-care and self-compassion** support you to allow and process your emotions?

Going Forward

1. How might you incorporate the Process outlined in this chapter to working with your emotions in your daily life?

2. How might focusing on just this first step of acknowledge, allow, accept assist you?

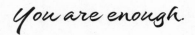

You are enough.

Chapter Six

Boundaries Part I
Values, Priorities and Goals

*"In absence of clearly defined goals, we become
strangely loyal to performing daily acts of trivia."*
—Author unknown

One of the reasons the boulder you are pushing feels so huge, daunting, and heavy is because you haven't taken the time to clarify what is truly important to you. Life can throw a lot your way, and if you're not careful, you can end-up pushing too much and spending time on things that do not reflect who you really are.

Determining Your Priorities and Goals
Will Allow You to Let Go

When we allow ourselves to be pulled in a million different directions, we can't become who we really are. We're too busy doing things that are not really us or ours to do. We are often left feeling overwhelmed and unfocused.

Part of identifying our values and priorities begins with noticing the cultural and internal pressures that drive us.

Women in particular tend to get trapped in *trying to do it all*. Society supports this behaviour, and we buy into it (which is our choice) because we receive a sense of value from it. Sometimes, we avoid prioritizing because choosing our priorities requires us to let go. Sometimes, we fear taking a step back from the things we do for others because we fear hurting our loved ones or losing our relationships. We may feel selfish or scared, but it is important to remember that as we *un* become, our relationships change. Becoming *you* means letting go of what no longer serves our highest calling or service. We can't become who we really are without first identifying what is us and is important to us.

Priorities, Goals and Boundaries

Priorities and goals provide clarity about your life now. From here, you set your boundaries around what your priorities and goals are, and then you begin to let the rest go.

Refer back to the very first exercise you did in the Introduction, about how you want your life to be. You may have written or drawn it out. As you think about this, consider what is really important for you right now. What matters to you at this place in your life? What do you really need right now? Is it more time, more calm, more peace, stronger family connections, stronger work connections? Take your time to really consider this.

Fear of Getting Clear

I have noticed that sometimes, women, myself included, resist identifying what is really important and making the decision to focus on only those things. We know that it can mean moving ahead, and we become fearful of what that would mean and the commitment it may take. We may fear being seen. Or we fear missing out on some things if we say *yes* to something else. We also worry about the people and things we may be saying *no* to.

We often justify our fear with thoughts like this: *If I don't think about what I want or where I want to head, I can ignore all of this and not face it.* The cost is that I ignore the prompts that keep telling me what is really me.

Thus, the boulder remains.

Confidence grows when we do the hard thing. It requires determined clarification which is part of the *un* becoming process.

What if Sisyphus had considered what was important to him and let the rest go? Although he had been assigned this boulder to push, and it appeared that he had no choice, perhaps he could have chosen to let go of what was holding him back and what was making that boulder so enormous. What if he knew, deep down, that he had choice and that not choosing was still a choice?

What if we acknowledged that much of what is heavy and enormous in our lives could really go? That we have a choice? How much lighter might we be?

The Process of Clarifying

When setting goals, many people leap right into what they want. When we do this, we miss the most important piece: the *why*. The feeling we want to achieve from the attainment of the goal is our *why*.

Why do you want to work less?

Why do you want to go into business for yourself?

Why do you want that new job?

Why do you want to travel?

Why do you want to do what you want to do?

The truth is that you want to achieve an experience and a feeling. Think about that for a moment. You may want to experience more excitement or adventure, a greater challenge, or more peace and calm. These, and other feelings, are what you are actually seeking.

Once you know what you want to feel, you can figure out what to do in order to feel it. It might mean starting your own business. It might mean finding a different job. It might mean working less—or working more. It might mean a lot of things. It might even mean doing fewer things here, and more things there, or stopping some things altogether. Start with the feeling of the *what* and the *how* will flow from there.

How we get it backwards

As an example, a lot of people going into entrepreneurship crave freedom and time for themselves and their families. Would they leave their high-paying jobs with benefits and financial security if they knew that they *might* lose their freedom along the way? Oftentimes, the path to entrepreneurship sees people become busier and busier, saying *yes* to everything and taking on too much. In retrospect, a structured, corporate life may have been what kept them on track. The lack of external structures may leave a person feeling overwhelmed, stressed out, and fatigued. If the person had identified, initially, how they wanted to feel, they may have found a different path to getting there and then been able to set boundaries around what they will do and won't do. Women tend to over-do.

Questions for Reflection

Journal your thoughts and take your time with each question to reflect, think, consider.

1. What do you want to *feel* and *experience* in the next six months to one year from now? For example, is it passion? Fun? Peace? Calm? Satisfaction? Joy? Excitement?

2. If you focused on creating a life around the feelings you want to experience, what activities do you imagine (a) being a part of and (b) not being a part of? Consider professional and the personal realm: for example, it may be more travel, more adventure, more down time, more recreation, more excitement, more education, less work, new work, more family time, less stress, less busy-ness, etc.

3. In order to create and serve the experience or feeling you desire, what might you need to remove from your life?

4. In order to create and serve the experience or feeling you desire what might you need to add to your life? Remember the feeling will guide you.

Determining what you want to feel and experience is essential to staying on your path, to achieving your goals, and becoming *you*. This is also an essential facet for setting boundaries. You get to choose what you want to have in your life and what you choose not to, which essentially protects your desire, the feeling and experience you want, your priorities and then your goals.

Exercise

Start by determining what you *value* at this point in your life. From there, pull out your main *priorities* to focus on. Once you determine your main priorities, you can design your *goals* and the following action steps.

Review

1. **Values**—what matters to you at your core; what shapes your purpose.

2. **Priorities**—what is most important to you right now in your life, determined by your values.

3. **Goals**—what you do to protect and develop your priorities; what is the action?

Now, it's time for you to determine what matters to you, right now, at this point in your life. You get to decide. Have fun with this.

Values Exercise

1. How do you want to experience your life? What is important to you now?

2. Based on Question 1, choose 10-15 values that are important to you at this time. You may have more than 15. You may have less.

Values List:

Achievement	Focus	Performance
Accuracy	Forward the action	Personal power
Acknowledgment	Free spirit	Pleasure
Advancement	Free time	Power
Adventure	Freedom	Precision
Aesthetics	Friendship	Productivity
Affection	Fun	Recognition
Authenticity	Growth	Responsibility
Autonomy	Happiness	Risk-taking
Balance	Integrity	Romance
Beauty	Independence	Security
Calm	Intellectual status	Self-expression
Caring	Health	Service
Challenge	Helping others	Spirituality
Change	Helping society	Stability
Clarity	Humor	Success
Contribution	Harmony	Tradition
Collaboration	Honesty	Trust
Community	Influence	Vitality
Compassion	Joy	Wealth
Connection	Knowledge	Wellness
Courage	Lack of pretense	Wisdom
Creativity	Leadership	Zest
Curiosity	Leisure	Add your own _____
Determination	Lightness	
Directness	Loyalty	
Ease	Love	
Economic security	Nurturing	
Elegance	Optimism	
Empowerment	Orderliness	
Excellence	Organization	
Excitement	Partnership	
Faith	Participation	
Family happiness	Peace	

(Portions of this exercise were adapted From: *Co-Active Coaching*. Whitworth, Kimsey-House; Sandahl)

Now, Identify and write down your three priorities

1. Once you have determined 10-15 values, group them and eliminate the ones that may not be as important right now. Next, write down *three* main categories, or three main themes. This will form your priorities. This is not an exact process. You may want to ask yourself what themes are emerging from your list. For example, it might be spirituality or personal growth, career, health/wellness, or family.

2. Once you have your three main priorities, consider, how much time and attention you are currently giving to each of them. Does your life reflect these priorities? As you look at your priorities, how does this feel to you? How is your mind responding? How is your body responding as you consider just these three priorities?

You may want to consider creating a *vision board* to reflect your three priorities. A vision board is essentially a visual representation of your goals. What do you want to experience in each of the areas you identified as priorities? The process of creating a vision board can also help you more clearly assess what is important to you. If you're interested in this, you can search for ideas and instructions online.

If a vision board doesn't interest you, still take the time to ask yourself: what are my three main priorities, and how will I protect and act on them?

Questions for Reflection Before Writing out Your Goals

1. What might you need to stop doing or remove from your life to focus on your three main priorities? Take some time to consider this. Write this out.

2. What do you need to start doing or add to your life to attend to your priorities?

3. How will focusing on these three priorities help create the feeling you want to experience?

4. How does it feel to have more clarity?

5. Review your values and your priorities. Is there anything you'd like to change or add?

Writing out your Goals and Intentions

It's important and helpful to write out what you want. Remember, you can adjust your goals at any time. Your goals serve your three main priorities. It's been said those who write down and imagine their goals accomplished are 1.2 to 1.4 times more likely to achieve them. What we write down, we are more likely to remember and consider important. Written or visual goals can be reviewed from time to time. You want to encode the goals into your brain, so that when you take the time to think about them, envision them, and feel what it would be like to achieve them, you are owning what you want to become.

Now that you're ready, read over the *goals* example following and then take your time *writing* out your goals.

A Template for Your Goals

Thinking about the next six months to one year, what do you want to do to help move you toward your three priorities? Your goals will center around these.

Goal: A goal is higher level. For example, perhaps one of your priorities is health and wellness and your goal may be: I want to reduce stress. Restate this in the positive. *I want to feel more peace and calm more consistently.* Your goal is simply re-stating one or more of your priorities in some manner.

How: What is the action you will commit to in order to achieve your goals? For example, with this same goal, *I want to feel more peace and calm,* here's what you may add to your life (these are the specific steps): (1) work through this workbook with a committed group of friends; (2) meet regularly; and (3) complete the exercises in between. Then, consider if there is anything you need to remove from your life and create action steps around that. For example, you may need to take less responsibility for others in some way. This is the *how,* the specific steps. As you begin to act, remind yourself of your goal to help you focus on those daily, weekly, and monthly action steps. Be sure to include how you will keep yourself accountable to working on your goals. Who might you check in with?

Now, write out your goals for this stage of your life. Make them realistic. Create action steps.

I recommend starting with two goals. You may find that it feels right for you to start with just one of these for now. You choose. Remember, action steps toward any goal can involve what needs to be removed, what you want to *stop* doing, what you will *start* doing, and how you will keep yourself accountable.

Goal #1:

_____

Specific Steps:

   1. _____

      • _____ (Sub steps)

      • _____

      • _____

   2. _____

   3. _____

Goal #2:

_____

Specific Steps:

   1. _____

   2. _____

   3. _____

As you review your goals, sit with them and notice how they feel. Do they fit? Do they feel heavy, scary, insurmountable, overwhelming? Or, do they feel light, encouraging and right? Feel it in your body. If it feels like too much, scale back. Perhaps there are fewer specific steps needed right now.

Once you've written out your goals, maybe you want to write your goals on something you can take with you, like a small card you laminate, a beautiful paper that you keep posted by your computer, or maybe a card to keep next to your phone. If you have created a vision board for your goals, have this in a place you see regularly. Review your goals from time to time and ask yourself: are these moving me forward? **Is anything overwhelming? What might I need to do more of? Less of?**

How does it feel to have more clarity about what is *you* for the next six months to one year?

When your goals are aligned with your priorities and your values, there is less push. When you're not pushing against yourself, you are in more flow. Clarifying what is best for you at this juncture in your life helps you determine what you can let go of, which is part of *un* becoming. This means letting go of what is not necessary, what is not healthy for you, and what may even be good, but isn't the best.

A beautiful benefit of this process is the risk you take. This process helps you strengthen your trust in yourself and *your* knowing of what is right for you.

Review Questions

Choose One or Two Questions to Discuss, Reflect on, and Journal:

1. Your values and priorities: what is most important for you right now in your life? Why do you think this is?

2. What are some of the changes you may need to make in your life to make these a priority?

3. Awareness: what may need to be removed from your life for you to focus on these priorities?

4. Awareness: what may need to be added to your life so that you can focus on these priorities?

5. What may get in the way of you living from your values and choosing to honor and act on your priorities?

6. How will focusing on these priorities help you move toward what you want in your life? How will this help you become more of who you really are?

7. What are one or more of your goals, and how do these support you and what you really want?

Summary

- The feeling and experiences you desire are the first step to determine who you are.

- Letting go of what is not right for you at this point in your life is uncomfortable, it takes courage, and it is part of *un* becoming.

- Once you set your three priorities, you can design your goals and then the corresponding action steps. This is clarity. Your goals are what you set boundaries on, which is what the next section is about.

Going Forward

Connecting and sharing with others

As you share with others, notice the expansion of your self-awareness. Notice the deepening connection to yourself and the connection to others that open sharing creates. We crave connection and, at the same time, we fear it because we fear being seen and rejected. Sharing with others takes courage, and as we share with supportive friends who are there for us, we open up more space within ourselves to expand and become more of who we really are. We feel more comfortable *un* becoming. The process of *un* becoming creates safety within yourself to become who you really are because you are noticing and facing what is hidden beneath the surface. Things like fear, when unaddressed, keep us from becoming who we really are. In this case, clearly identifying what we want and how we want to get there will help us take one step closer to our goals.

Self-Care and Self-Compassion Don't Go Away

Continue to notice how your practices of self-care (I recommend at least one practice daily) and self-compassion (allowing and acknowledging what you feel, speaking kindly to yourself) support you in *un* becoming, and as you consider acting on your goals.

Keep your goals alive to keep your dreams alive!

You are enough.

Chapter Seven

Boundaries Part II
Let's Dive In

"As you start to walk on the way, the way appears."
—Rumi

Un becoming involves setting boundaries. It involves letting go of things that you have been choosing, but do not serve your three main priorities and your highest purpose. It is letting go of unrealistic expectations for yourself, of focusing on others to your detriment, and of trying to be perfect or people-please or over-achieve.

Boundaries are the framework you erect in your life to help protect your time management, your relationships, your health and wellness, and the pursuit of your dreams.

Boundaries are the line that you draw around you: your life, your values, your priorities and your goals.

My Journey with Boundaries

Over thirty years of sitting across from women of all ages and listening to them share intimate details about their lives and struggles, it became apparent to me that women struggle with boundaries. It's also apparent when they wind their way through finding and setting boundaries, and then start saying yes to the right things, they become who they really are. This is the power of boundaries.

Learning about boundaries was life-changing for me: it allowed me to courageously step into my life and let go of other people's expectations of me. I realized that I needed to stop blaming others and take responsibility for my over-achieving and people-pleasing. I realized this at a point in my life when I was exhausted from doing too much and taking on unrealistic expectations (from others and myself).

At my worst, I could barely carry on a conversation with someone without tearing up. I was tired and stressed, wired, and unable to sleep as my busy mind kept thinking about everything I still had to do and how I wasn't measuring up. When I finally did take an extended leave from work, I began to reflect on what needed to change.

I realized that I had been taught about and I readily embraced service to others, but never about considering my own wellbeing or health. I knew about pushing, but I did not know about self-care and boundaries, like slowing down and saying "no." I wasn't even considering this. It actually seemed wrong.

During my time off, I tried to rest and relax, although most of the time my mind was busy being critical of myself and others. However, I began to consider what I needed to do differently. When I returned to work, I was determined to do things differently, and I did. I requested more help. I started to take better care of my own well-being and I stopped working long hours. I faced the fact that others might think I was being irresponsible or wasn't very capable (a big fear of mine), and I needed to face this fear. This was a pivotal point in my life, the recognition that I am responsible for my time, my work, and my well-being.

I started to have more conversations about what I could and couldn't do in my work. Saying no rocked the boat. This made me notice that there was an underlying drive behind my over-doing and people-pleasing: an almost desperate need to be respected and liked by others, especially those in authority. It was so powerful that in my efforts to meet those needs, I had ignored *me*. I also realized that others benefit from my poor boundaries, which makes over-doing a challenge to let go of. Others might take advantage of that.

My need to please was not about other people or how much I cared about them. My need to please was about *me*. I was trying to manipulate my life in a way that garnered respect and adoration of other people. This was my way of trying to stay in control, and it caused me a lot of distress. This was a huge *un* becoming stage for me. I was letting go of people-pleasing and over-achieving. In other words, I was unravelling and letting go of the belief that I didn't have value unless I was over-achieving or pleasing everyone around me. I had been so afraid of disappointing others that I became exhausted and over-whelmed.

Once I started working on these limiting beliefs, I began to set boundaries with myself and others. I determined first what I wanted to feel. Peace and calm. I then began sorting through what I needed to bring into my life and what I needed to discard. Understanding and implementing boundaries changed my life. But it wasn't easy.

This is what I learned from setting boundaries:

- I had to learn to accept other people's disappointment and/or anger at times when I needed to say no or ask for what I needed. The boundaries were not always with other people, but often with myself. This could mean choosing to take time for my own health and overall wellness, to exercise, to go out with friends, or to have a social life. To do this, I needed to create time and space, which meant that I needed a boundary to work less and protect my time.

- I had to deal with my own guilt when I slowed down, took care of myself, and said *no*. The voices in my head were very loud at first. *They won't like you. They will think you are lazy. They will think you don't care about others. They will talk about you negatively to others. You will disappoint them. You are being selfish! You're too self-focused! You are being mean. What about all the people who need your help? You're being irresponsible!* I did feel guilty. It was challenging, but I kept up with the path of setting boundaries.

- I had to take care of myself first. I discovered that it was my job to care of myself, not in a *no one else cares about me* way, but in a new way. I needed to take responsibility for the beliefs, behaviour and feelings that I had not been aware of before. In order to set boundaries, I needed to see why I was over-achieving and people-pleasing. This is so important to understand. It released me from expecting others to know what I want or need, or to take care of me. This was my responsibility.

- I had to take responsibility for where I was at and how I got there. I had to stop blaming others for asking me to do things and expecting me to work long hours, or for asking me to do more. I had to wake up to this fundamental truth: I had a choice, and my previous choices had gotten me where I was. And if that was the case, then my new beliefs and choices could get me out of this spot, too.

- I learned that I was engaging in people-pleasing, perfectionism, and over-achieving, all at once. I believed that my value relied on what people thought of me. As I became aware of this, the insight became a relief to me because I knew I could change how I believed and behaved. I could start to believe that I had value regardless, of what others thought of me. I took action. I upped my self-care, and I reduced my work time.

Things to Remember About Boundaries

- Boundaries are action. The choices you make to protect you and your life goals, desires and dreams are *setting* boundaries.

- What you've done in the past may not work now. Remember that metaphor about going around the mountain? If we don't set boundaries and make different choices in our best interest, we will keep going around the mountain and come back to the same place. Going around the mountain is avoidance. If you don't set boundaries now, you will need to set them later. Setting boundaries will help you go through the mountain and help you break old patterns by facing your life and taking action to change it.

- Setting boundaries means that you're going into the underworld. You begin to see, face, and deal with what is beneath the surface. Your limiting beliefs like *I have to be perfect, I have to be nice, I have to be successful*, will show up. You feel the discomfort and guilt as you begin to see why you have been doing what you have been doing and the limiting beliefs driving your poor boundaries. When you go *through* the mountain and begin to care for yourself, you start to unravel what keeps you from being you.

What if Sisyphus had considered boundaries? Since boundary setting starts with pausing and determining how you feel, Sisyphus would have needed to start here. Sisyphus kept pushing, and all he could see was the boulder in front of him. I can only imagine how discouraged and frustrated he must've felt each time the boulder rolled back after such enormous effort. It truly was an uphill battle for him. Does this sound familiar? This is where many women find themselves at some point in their lives: frustrated, discouraged, and worn out from an uphill battle. If Sisyphus had paused and reflected on what he felt, he may have realized the futility of his actions. Maybe there are boulders we are pushing, but don't need to?

Question for Reflection—Part I

Review each of the following areas and journal your thoughts about them. Consider whether you are nurturing and protecting yourself in each of these areas:

1. **Mental:** Are you feeling overwhelmed, unfocused, or distracted? Do you engage in self-criticism? Is your mind busy and full of to do lists, what you should have done, etc? How well do you nourish your mental wellness?

2. **Physical:** Are you physically tired, ill, not sleeping, and/or showing stress-related symptoms like headaches, muscle aches and pains, heart problems, or high blood pressure? How well do you nourish your physical health?

3. **Emotional:** Do you feel resentful, angry, impatient, irritable, and over-stressed? How well do you nourish your emotional health?

4. **Spiritual:** Are you experiencing a sense of loss or a lack of direction or purpose? Are you feeling spiritually alone or disconnected from a higher source? How well are you nourish your spiritual life?

5. **Relationships:** How healthy are your important relationships? Are the most important people getting your time? How well are you nourishing your important relationships?

6. **Goals, Dreams, Life Purpose:** What have you put on hold? What are you willing to believe in for yourself? How well are you nourishing your goals and dreams?

Why Don't Women Say *No* in Order to Say *Yes* to Themselves?

You can have all the plans you want, all the ideas and dreams you want, but you need to set boundaries in order to become who you really are. Ask yourself: why do so many women struggle with setting boundaries? Why do you?

Questions for Reflection—Part II

Review the five areas below and consider how these impact how you create boundaries.

1. **Cultural pressure and expectations:** Women are taught to be nice, which can impact our willingness to be boldly truthful. Second, as society changes, women are doing more. More opportunities outside of the home and more opportunities in career and work means more in our lives. How does saying yes to your future challenge how you set boundaries?

2. **Perfectionism:** Many women work more to reach an unspoken degree of perfection. Perfectionism keeps us from making a real connection with our work and others, and makes us feel worse, not better. How might perfectionism be impacting your boundaries?

3. **People-pleasing and fear of conflict:** Research supports that we are biologically different than men when it comes to conflict. Louann Brizendine, author of *The Female Brain*, says that "the female brain has a far more negative reaction to relationship conflict and rejection than does the male brain... In women, conflict is more likely to set in motion a cascade of negative chemical (brain) reactions, creating feelings of stress, upset and fear." She explains that when a relationship is threatened or lost, serotonin, dopamine and endorphins drop dramatically, and cortisol, the stress hormone, takes over. When feelings get hurt, a hormonal shift happens. Combine that with the fact that a woman's self-esteem is partly maintained by the ability to sustain intimate relationships, and it is no wonder we are stressed when we consider saying *no*

and hurting someone's feelings! How might a need to please and/or a fear of conflict be impacting your boundaries?

4. **Over-Achievement:** The drive to be more successful can keep many women in an endless pursuit of more. But at what cost? This drive is motivated by a sense of not being enough. How might over-achievement be impacting your boundary setting?

5. **Being Enough:** As we have seen, being there for others can give us a false sense of self-worth. Eventually, we feel empty, maybe even worse. How might the pursuit of *being enough* be affecting your boundaries?

Four Key Areas Impacted by Boundaries

Your Time, Relationships, Health and Wellness and Dreams

Protect and Manage Your Time

Note the emphasis on *your* time because this is *your* responsibility, not anyone else's. It is *your* time, so *you* decide what is best and right for you at any moment.

This is where I started—realizing that my time was my choice. Many of us do way too much to take care of way too many people. Not only do we over-tax ourselves, but we sometimes enable others—even our children, colleagues, and spouses—to avoid responsibility.

Many women wait for other people to understand before they start changing themselves. If you wait for others to give you the go-ahead, you let others choose for you. It is *you* who decides, and when you choose, you build your core resilient strength. Choosing also builds your confidence.

Right now, you may be living in a way that says that your time is not your own. You might be allowing others to decide for you to keep the peace. But when you say "yes" to one more responsibility out of obligation, you're the one who lives with the consequences—whether it is stress, exhaustion, or feeling overwhelmed.

Protect and Enhance Your Relationships

What kind of people do you want in your inner circle? What are your criteria? Here are mine:

- Interesting people;
- Those I can learn from and who help me grow;
- People who respect me and have my back;
- People who support me and listen to me;
- People who are honest and trustworthy.

What is your criteria for your inner-circle?

Protect Your Health and Wellness

One of the most detrimental things about poor boundaries is the kind of harm you do to yourself by *ignoring* yourself. This goes way beyond physical, mental, and emotional stress. It is not just that you wear and stress yourself out, or that you don't take care of yourself emotionally, physically, mentally or spiritually. The problem is also that these decisions have not been yours—they have been your default. You have done it to please or appease others. You have done it because you felt obligated. This is a *yes* out of fear, not love. It is fear of disappointing, or fear of not being enough that hurts your self-esteem and self-respect. You aren't just making poor choices—you are ignoring *yourself*. This, in my opinion, is one of the worst kinds of abuse.

Protect and Pursue Your Dreams

Boundaries protect your goals and dreams. They help you say *no* to the unnecessary, so that you can say *yes* to your dreams (yourself).

How to Set Boundaries and Say No

Now that you've reviewed the importance of boundaries and the main areas they affect, let's take a look at how to set them. This requires concentrated focus and determination. This is where we just need to do it, regardless of how nervous or fearful we are.

A. **Learn to listen to yourself, your thoughts, your emotions and your body.**

By doing so, we can wake up to what we really want and who we truly are.

For example, one of my clients had an upcoming job interview, so I asked:

"What are you feeling?"

She didn't really know.

"Is there anything showing up in your body? Any feeling?"

She stopped and paid attention. She noticed that her chest was tight and stressed, and that her stomach was in a bit of a knot.

We explored the emotions behind this. She admitted that she was feeling nervous about accepting this work and nervous about the possibility of not accepting it.

We explored each worry separately, starting with why she may not want to accept this work.

She determined that although the job was a good one, given everything else going on in her life, it may not be the right timing. It might be too much. She also recognized that although she liked the work, it was not her primary love. Her body was telling her the truth. Your body doesn't lie. Once she realized that some of the tightness in her chest had to do with being overwhelmed and that this work may not be her main love, she acknowledged this, and the tightness eased. The tightness eased when she considered saying no to the work.

We then explored why she was feeling nervous about not taking the job. She said she was afraid of missing out. People were telling her that this was a great opportunity.

Once she accepted this fear and realized that it was okay (reframing) even if she *did* miss out, she was more able to let this fear go. When she thought about saying *no* to this opportunity, *we checked in with her body again.*

She was feeling more relaxed. She still felt somewhat nervous about declining the offer, but she was able to move ahead more confidently. Once she fully accepted what her body was telling her, the feeling behind it, and the *why* of the feeling, she was able to be more decisive about her decision. This decision became her boundary. She had more clarity on why her decision was a *no, not now* and she felt less guilt as a result.

An interesting aspect about her journey is that once she said *no* to this opportunity, she had much more time to focus on what she was truly passionate about. Saying "no" to something that was good, but not *quite* right for her created the time and space for her to move into work that was really *hers.* Her creativity and success soared.

It takes courage to say *no* to good things when we have not yet experienced the *what's next* that could be great. Our bodies speak to us quickly. It may take some practice to slow down and tune in. We need to slow down to pause and reflect, and this takes courage.

Sometimes, we don't know what we are feeling. We have trouble naming it. If this is you, you are not alone (and you can refer to Chapter Five on Emotions). But you can check in with your body, just like this woman did.

B. **Have a clear decision-making process.**

Consider the following questions to help you make decisions.

1. Is this necessary and if so, does it need to be done right now?

2. Is this any of my business? Am I stepping into someone else's boundary?

3. Does this fit with my present priorities? (Refer to the priorities you identified in Chapter Six).

4. How do I feel? What is this about? What do I need? What will I do? Go back to the steps in processing emotions in Chapter Five.

   - What do you feel? Where do you feel it? Acknowledge and accept the feeling. Stay with the feeling and allow it. Accept it.

   - Ask yourself: what is this feeling about?

   - What do you need?

   - Decide what to do based on what you feel and need. Is a conversation needed? Do you need to set a boundary with someone or yourself? Do you need to do less or to let go of something?

C. **Review your priorities from Chapter 3.**

Does this decision align with your priorities?

D. **Revisit your goals from the last chapter**.

Review your goals. How are your boundaries protecting your goals?

E. **Practice saying *no*.**

F. **Accept your feelings when you say *no***. You will likely feel guilt, shame, or regret (especially if you're setting boundaries in new areas of your life). Be prepared for these feelings but know that most of it is false guilt.

Exercise—Practicing Boundary-Setting

Take some time to work through a situation or challenge that you are presently experiencing. If you can't think of one right now, think of a challenging situation in the past. Try to work through the process outlined above. Take your time.

As you start to set boundaries, it may be awkward. You may worry about coming across as aggressive. You may stumble over your words or falter. You are learning. You are experimenting. If you do notice aggression, simply apologize, learn, and move on.

Make a few changes at a time. Choose what is manageable. This may be one change at a time.

I have the privilege of working with women who have become clear about who they are and what their purpose is.

They have let go of what is not them, and they continue to do so—not perfectly, but they do it. This didn't happen overnight, but rather through thoughtful reflection and brave action.

They have un become in order to become their real selves.

They have become more resilient to others' disappointment.

They have become more self-compassionate, and they are more relaxed.

They have time for their own pursuits.

They are sometimes angry, overwhelmed, and unfocused. They are human with feelings, just like you and I.

Questions for Reflection

1. How might self-compassion support you in setting boundaries?

2. How do any of your limiting beliefs (perfectionism, people-pleasing and over-achieving) affect your boundary setting?

3. How do you think that being aware of your feelings can help you set boundaries?

Boundaries Summary

Living your own life means owning it and not allowing others' or your own unrealistic expectations make you choose unhealthy boundaries.

Remember:

- You are accountable for your own life. Therefore, you are responsible for setting and keeping your boundaries.

- Stay out of other people's boundaries—respect their *no* too.

- Pay attention to your instincts and feelings about things or people—these help you know your boundaries and protect you.

- Develop your *no* muscle. Set limits. Realize that you have a limited amount of time, money, and energy.

- Become proactive rather than reactive. People with boundary issues are often not the initiators, and they can let things happen *to* them rather than taking initiative and responsibility for their own choices.

- Review your priorities and goals. Your boundaries protect and honor your priorities and goals. That is the purpose of boundaries.

- Just do it. Say no to what you don't want. Say yes to what you do want.

Boundaries—Questions for Reflection

Choose 1-2 questions below, reflect and journal your thoughts and insights.

1. Write out all your thoughts about boundaries and why you think they are important for you.

2. Boundaries are compassionate and respectful, both to yourself and others. Reflect on a time when you set a boundary. How was this compassionate and respectful to you and the other person?

3. Consider how you could become kinder and firmer when setting boundaries.

4. In the next chapter, we will be discussing courageous conversations. How might holding other people accountable (setting boundaries) actually be respectful and kind?

5. What areas of your life and/or relationships are you tolerating right now? What might you do to shift this?

6. Are there any other steps that you could take to strengthen your goals? (Hint: It might be doing less or removing something from your to-do list.) What will you do?

7. Reflect on the key areas that your boundaries protect. How might you enhance your boundaries in each area?

a. Time management

b. Relationships

c. Your own health and wellness

d. Your dreams and goals

Going Forward

As you courageously set boundaries, you will *un* become. you will unravel those beliefs and behaviours that get in the way of being the real *you*. In fact, setting boundaries is one of the most powerful ways to support your *un* becoming. This is part of a new way of living and being. You will feel more refreshed, more free.

Consider experimenting with boundaries. Boundaries are not something you do against someone or a situation. That is pushing. Setting boundaries is something you do for yourself. As you move forward with boundaries, consider experimenting. This will allow you more freedom to practice and play with boundary setting as boundaries are not always 100% clear or a straight line. Give yourself the freedom to do this imperfectly. This is self-compassion in action. Boundaries is the 'only' way to protect you, and what is important to you so you can become who you really are.

"Your new life is going to cost you your old one. It's going to cost you your comfort zone and your sense of direction. It's going to cost you relationships and friends. It's going to cost you being liked and understood. But it doesn't matter. Because the people who are meant for you are going to meet you on the other side. And you're going to build a new comfort zone around the things that actually move you forward. And instead of being liked, you're going to be loved. Instead of being understood, you're going to be seen. All you're going to lose is what was built for a person you no longer are. Let it go."
—Brianne West, The Minds Journal

You are enough.

Chapter Eight

Courageous Connection

"When you follow the crowd you lose yourself but when you follow your soul you will lose the crowd. Eventually your soul tribe will appear. But do not fear the process of solitude."
—Amazonian Dictum

What Are Courageous Connections?

Courageous connection involves courageous conversations to clarify who we are with others. To *un* become, we must face our relationships and who *we* are, in those relationships. Sometimes, we need to clear up what's not working. Sometimes, we need to lovingly let go. We want to treat ourselves with kindness and respect, and we want to make sure others do too. Sometimes, we need to be more vulnerable with those we love. We almost always need to deepen our ability to listen. Sisyphus led a lonely existence, as his pushing was a solitary affair: there was no connection with others. Perhaps this led to him to more pushing. He was shut off. He wasn't aware of what he could do differently, and he had no one to talk to about his troubles. He had no one to share the load. Our relationships can and will help us to pause and see what we are pushing or tolerating. They can provide support and insight into how we are feeling. Talking to others can and will bring deeper insights and awareness. Others almost always help us become more courageous in doing the work of *un* becoming, and we can do the same for others.

To create courageous connections, we need to understand and practice three things:

1. Conversations—A courageous conversation is needed when there's been a challenge with our boundaries.

2. Vulnerability—A courageous connection requires being vulnerable with those we trust.

3. Deep Listening—A courageous connection requires deep listening.

The Neurochemistry of Connection

Positive interactions with others release our feel-good hormones: oxytocin, serotonin, and endorphins. When we connect with others and feel listened to, understood, and valued, we feel better. We also feel better when we do the same for others. This happens, in part, because of the release of these chemicals. Research shows that oxytocin can contribute to feelings of trust, empathy, affection, and stability. Serotonin is our feel-good neurotransmitter, and it is released when we feel understood, valued and connected. Endorphins create a strong sense of pleasure, which provides resistance to pain and loss. Connecting with others supports us by decreasing the stress in our body. As women, we crave connection. Our body loves it. Women truly thrive in healthy and supportive relationships.

Evaluate your present relationships

Our relationships can help us to *un* become. Some are supportive and healthy. Some need some attention. Some provide challenges by triggering our false beliefs and bringing our awareness to them. We start to notice things that allow us to make healthier choices. As we begin to look closely, beneath the surface, we may notice things that need to change a little, or a lot.

Questions for Reflection

1. Draw a small circle on a plain piece of paper (or in your journal) about the size of the bottom of a glass or mug. Draw another circle around that one, allowing about 2 inches of space between each one. Then draw a third circle around that, again about 2 inches wider than the previous circle.

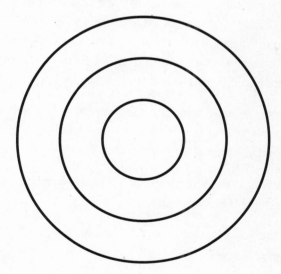

2. Next, consider your three relationship levels: the first is your inner circle, those you feel closest to and trust the most. The second circle is the next relationship level, and it includes those you may

like and spend time with, but who are not as important to you as those in your inner circle. The last circle is all the other people that are in your life in some manner—your acquaintances, people you work with, etc. Begin to fill in these circles with the names of the people in your circles.

3. As you review those who are in your circles, rate each of the first and second circle relationships on a scale of 0-10 (10 means that you are fully satisfied and happy in that relationship and 0 means that you are not at all satisfied, and perhaps distressed about it.) Leave the third circle for now. Don't overthink it, just go with your gut instinct.

4. As you review the names and the ratings in your inner and then your second circle, what do you notice? Are there some relationships that are not as healthy as you would like?

5. When you consider the third circle, review the importance of these relationships. Are you giving any of these more time and attention than those in your inner or second circle? If so, consider what you might want to change. Sometimes, we give more attention and care to acquaintances than we do our own inner circle. Sometimes, we take our inner circle for granted.

6. As you review the relationships in your inner and second circle, consider the following questions. Invite yourself to play with this and journal your insights.

   - Are there any relationships that need to be in a different circle? If so, move them.

   - Are you pleased with the number of relationships in each circle?

   - What might you be tolerating in any of these relationships?

- What might you be doing or not doing that contributes to the challenges or weakened connection in this relationship?

- Are there any relationships you need to let go of, or step back from?

- Next, take a closer look at the relationship(s) you would like to enhance by strengthening the connection. How might you do that?

The Three Steps of Courageous Connections

The First Piece: Courageous Conversations

Courageous conversations are compassionately truthful, and truthfully compassionate.

Courageous conversations require speaking the truth and doing so respectfully. It requires respecting your needs and others'. This can be complicated because being human means experiencing complexity. It is possible to have genuine and supportive conversations, even during conflict and tense times. These conversations are necessary for a full, healthy life: mentally, emotionally, spiritually and physically. These conversations offer us an opportunity to deepen connection, instead of diminishing it—as we may fear.

To enhance a connection, you may need a courageous conversation.

For the relationships you want to enhance, consider what you may need to address. We'll talk about how to do that in a moment. For now, take your time to reflect on what you need or desire. Write in your journal.

- You want to spend more time with this person.

- You want this person to respect you more.

- You want this relationship to be more balanced.

- You want them to listen to you more deeply.

- You want to feel more understood.

- You want more emotional connection.

- You want less drama.

- You want time or space.

- You want to do less.

- You want to do different things.

- Anything else?

Taking a Closer Look at Courageous Conversations

A courageous conversation is simply a conversation you have with someone who said or did something, or didn't say or didn't do something, that was problematic for you. These could be one time behaviors or behaviors that happen over a period of time.

The purpose of a courageous conversation is to protect the priorities you reflected on and considered in Chapter Six. If you don't know what you want in your life, you won't know what to be assertive about or what to ask for. Consider your priorities and your goals once again. A courageous conversation is simply one way you communicate your boundaries.

A courageous conversation is assertive. Assertive action is communicating clearly about behaviour that is not acceptable. Assertiveness takes care of issues and challenges more quickly. Being assertive does not let negativity build up.

Courageous conversations can be challenging. Here are some of the things that may get in the way of a productive courageous conversation:

- Women tend to fear reprisal, so our limiting desires (to please, to not rock the boat, to appear perfect, to over-achieve) can get in the way of saying what needs to be said.

- We fear that others might see our vulnerabilities and reject us.

- We question ourselves and often lean toward just letting it go instead of dealing with it.

- We may become defensive, withdrawn, or lash out instead of respectfully and calmly having a conversation.

- We may not listen well, or others might not listen well, and either side may interpret the conversation as an attack on them.

- We are still practicing how to say what we need to with clarity and respect. We may say too much or too little, or a disrespectful tone may creep into our way of speaking.

- Other people may not want us to be assertive.

The following are the steps toward planning and executing a courageous conversation.

The Steps of a Courageous Conversation

Preparation: Consider writing out your goals for this conversation. What would you like to happen? Is your goal to improve the relationship? To clear up a concern? Something else?

Remember, the conversation should show respect to you and the other person. Remind yourself that it is compassionate to clarify and hold people accountable for their behaviours. Remember what we learned about emotions, here. Those steps can help you reflect on how you feel, why you feel that, what you need, and what you will do.

From here, there are three core steps to follow in a Courageous Conversation.

Step 1. The situation: In one sentence, clearly and concisely communicate what was said or done.

Step 2. The impact on you, or others and why: Communicate the impact you experienced. It's important to include how you felt then and/or how you feel now, and why—be sure to use feeling words (remember Chapter Five—Emotions).

Use feeling words instead of saying things like, "*I was disrespected,*" or "*you were unprofessional*". These are not descriptive of how you feel. It's important to share the emotional impact on you, as this provides the opportunity for the other person to not only acknowledge and take responsibility for what they did, but also to acknowledge how it affected you. If you use non feeling words, like *disrespected,* the other person may become defensive which has the potential to derail the conversation.

It might sound more like, "*What you said hurt my feelings*", or "*What you did left me feeling helpless and confused.*"

Also provide a brief description of why you feel as you do.

If and when they do acknowledge how what they said or did made you feel, you will be understood. Keep your statement simple—going into too much detail can confuse the conversation.

Step 3. What you would like to happen, and what do you need going forward? After some discussion (if needed), be very clear, with descriptive behavioural words, about what you expect or need going forward. Don't be vague. Get a commitment from the other person, if possible. This is the accountability part. If they acknowledge that what they did impacted you, then you are also responsible for holding them accountable. You may need to remind them when they slip.

Exercise

Think of a situation that you may have been tolerating and write out what you would say to the other individual to change that situation, using the three steps above. This may be the same situation or challenge you worked through in the Boundaries chapter, or it may be a different one. Create one sentence for each statement. You may need to spend some time writing out the entire situation first so you can determine the specific behaviour that was problematic. You may also need to talk this through with an objective party.

Example:

1. **Step 1:** *"Yesterday in the meeting, when you said, 'you never complete anything on time'* (Clear, behavioural, and to the point.)

2. **Step 2:** *I was embarrassed because this was said in front of others. I also felt confused because I'm not sure what you are referring to.* (Note the use of "feeling words": *embarrassed* and *confused*, accompanied by the "why.")

3. **Step 3:** *"Can we talk about this?"* After the discussion, be sure to gain clarity about what you expect in the future. You may want to say something like, *"Going forward, please discuss your concerns with me privately and provide examples of what you mean."* You need to be clear about your specific wants and needs.

Now, consider your situation and work through the steps below as you write out your thoughts.

How to Prepare for a Courageous Conversation:

1. Write out as much about the situation as possible ahead of time. Take your time. Review your notes.

2. Determine what the issue or problem is. Determine how you felt or feel. Determine what your specific needs are.

3. Prepare and write out what you plan to say to the other person. This is the core of the conversation:

   a. **The situation**. Create one sentence that describes the situation clearly and succinctly, with no blame of the other person. You are describing behaviours.

   b. **How you feel and why**. Create one sentence that describes the emotional impact on you. How did you feel? How do you still feel? Remember to use *feeling words* instead of expressions like *"you treated me disrespectfully."* This can be one of the hardest parts of this conversation.

   c. **What you would like to see happen/what do you need?** Be clear ahead of time. What are you prepared for? Remember, they may want to negotiate. Create one statement that describes what you would like to see or what you need going forward. This needs to be behavioural and measurable. For example, what does more respect actually look like?

4. Plan your request to have a conversation. Consider something like, *"I'd like to talk to you about our conversation yesterday. When would be a good time?"* Don't give too many details, just enough for them to know the context.

5. Plan what you will say to start the conversation. This should clearly demonstrate why you are having this conversation. Here's an example: *"I'd like to talk to you about our conversation yesterday because our relationship is important to me."* Then, invite them to

participate with a question: *"Would you be willing to allow me to share my perspective?"*

6. Review your initial set-up statements, your conversation-starter statement, and then the core statements (i.e., the 3 steps) with someone who isn't involved in the situation and ask for feedback. Use the following questions to determine the clarity and respect of your statements:

7. Are you clear about the problem or issue, the impact on you, and what you need going forward?

8. Did you use one sentence for each of the three steps? Did you follow all the guidelines for each step?

9. Did you use feeling words to describe the impact on you? Did you use just one or two emotion words?

10. Are you respectful with your words and tone?

11. Roleplay with someone you trust. This helps to prepare you by getting you into the realness of the conversation.

12. Have the conversation.

13. At the end of the conversation, be sure to get a commitment from them as to how their behaviour will change moving forward.

14. Review. Take some time to review on your own: What went well? What would you do differently? Take some time to applaud yourself. Is there anything that still needs to be said? How did the other person respond? These conversations are not easy, and they require a lot of emotional and mental energy. You did it!

Other Things to Consider Before You have the Conversation

· **What will the outcome be?** If this situation were resolved, what could be the benefit(s) to you? To them? To others?

- **Take care of your emotions first.** Think about the situation, feel what you feel, and acknowledge what you feel. Move from blame (*The other person is a terrible human being for doing this*) or shame (*I'm a terrible human being for not being able to handle this*) to acceptance. This will help you create a more open, safe, and respectful space to have a conversation.

- **Let go of the outcome**. Know how you want this to go, what you want to say, how you want to say it, and what you would like to achieve. Think about the best possible outcome. Even imagine it. Then, let go of any need for the other person to agree or understand. That is not in your control. Hope for the best but let go of any expected outcome. In your mind, know that you will do your best to do your part, and that alone is success. Encourage yourself. This is courageous. Think about and prepare for the worst possible outcome as well.

- **Prepare for distractions and/or side tracking**. Consider that the other individual may bring up other issues, deflect, or get defensive. Prepare for this, and plan to use a statement like, *"That's a good point, let's talk about that next."* Then, get back to your conversation. This holds them accountable for what they say, and you are respectful for acknowledging it. It also allows you to stay on track with the subject at hand.

- **Invite them to share any concerns they have with you.** You may need to set up another time to have this conversation.

Conversations Are for Connection

Remember, the conversation is about creating an emotionally safe environment to allow for connection between you and the other party for honesty to occur. Often, this is only the first step toward setting and communicating boundaries. You may need to follow up with them and provide feedback on how they are doing.

Stop Being SO Nice Doesn't Mean Don't BE Nice

If your goal is to be perfect or nice, you will have trouble being assertive. Focusing on being nice will put your true connection at risk. *Stop being SO nice,* means stop making *nice* your only priority. If your actual priorities are being pushed aside, it is important that you are assertive. I love to see how courageous and assertive conversations help women build their confidence. They finally face the things they have feared for so long. They also build their 'no' muscle (boundaries) and they begin to act on and trust themselves. This builds confidence.

Go for Assertive, not Aggressive

Of course, a true connection can't happen when there is aggressive behaviour. Aggressiveness diminishes connection. People feel unsafe. Sometimes, as women, we are angry and dump our anger onto someone else or verbally attack because we believe that we have a right to. The truth is, you can and will feel hurt, angry, resentful, mad, disappointed or sad, but dumping that onto another person is aggressive, not assertive. Aggressive communication may come from a place of feeling you're not enough. You get defensive out of a need for self-protection.

Aggressive is different than *assertive.* Whereas being assertive requires clear, direct communication, being aggressive may involve a harsh tone. Aggressive communication may involve name calling or shaming; (i.e. "*You always do this.*" or "*You'll never be good enough for this.*") Aggression also manifests as sarcasm, or verbal attacks. Sometimes, assertion gets labelled aggressive when it's not. If that happens, it isn't your fault. But take the time to ask yourself whether some aggression is bleeding into your assertion.

If your style is to be more aggressive, you will create unsafe relationships. People will fear you, and they won't feel confident being themselves. They will withdraw. You won't be able to experience a real connection with them because you won't have provided the safety for them to be themselves and be honest. Aggressiveness communicates the need or desire to control a situation. Aggressiveness may be a form of self-protection because it holds people at arms-length.

Although aggressiveness can look or feel like confidence, it is essentially power over someone or something, and it comes from a place of fear. Telling others what to do, or providing a solution they haven't asked for, is also aggressive. It diminishes trust. For many women, fixing others, rather than trusting others to navigate their journey, is a pattern. Fixing is a form of aggression.

Passive Connection Isn't Real Connection

Passivity can take many forms.

- Passivity is letting others make decisions that should be yours. This is dependence, not independence. It will hurt you, your health, and other people as well.

- Passivity may make you over-apologize, or apologize when it's not needed.

- Passivity may make you ask for permission when permission is not needed. Consider the impact on others if you do this. Healthy people don't want control over you or your choices. They just want to know your truth.

Passive behaviour and communication also decrease connection because it's not honest. To say *"it's okay"* when it's not is passive. If you are passive, your path will get cluttered with unnecessary things, situations, work, responsibilities, relationships, and critical thoughts that deplete your energy and keep you from living a full, inspired life. In short, passive behaviour prevents you from *un* becoming, and therefore it prevents you from becoming *you*.

Passivity is also a form of control. By being passive, we are trying to control others' responses. By giving in and being overly nice or overly helpful, we are trying to control the other person so that they like us, or so they are not disappointed in us. Passivity is also based in fear—fear of what others will think of you, say about you, and feel toward you. Passivity gives more power to others and, as a result, it decreases true connection. It creates unequal relationships.

Passive behaviour makes you withhold necessary information. Withholding is a passive form of lying, which makes it impossible for people to trust you. Being passive can also look like relying on others to make your life better.

Passive women sometimes meddle. It's true. Sometimes women can be so uncomfortable with other people's pain that they try to fix it. As a result, they get in the way of the other person's process, journey, or choices. Fixing does not feel good to others, and they may experience it as aggression. Sometimes, passive people have not learned to tolerate strong or reactionary emotion in others, and this can lead to aggressive behaviour on their part

Remember, assertiveness is neither passivity or aggression. It means allowing others to have their own journey. It means respectfully speaking your truth.

Passive-Aggression Is a Problem Too

Passive-aggressive behaviour or communication is another attempt at control in an indirect way, and it diminishes real connection. An attempt to communicate something without being clear and direct may be considered passive-aggressive. It is behaviour that is outwardly passive, yet inwardly aggressive.

An example may be saying *"I'm fine,"* while your tone and body language indicates otherwise. Another example might be showing up late because the other person *deserves* it. It is refusing to talk to, and/

or ignoring, someone who is open and willing to discuss concerns, simply because you are angry at them.

Passive-aggressive behaviour is silent sabotage. It's an indirect way to control, without demonstrating the courage to address something directly. Other examples may be, sighing, rolling eyes, using sarcasm, slamming doors, or even talking behind someone's back. The point is always the motive. If it's an indirect way to communicate your hurt, anger, frustration, or disappointment without directly conversing about it, it is likely passive-aggressive.

Questions for Reflection

Consider the first three questions, which review aggressiveness, passivity, and passive aggressiveness.

1. Where might you be **aggressive**—pushy, controlling, bossy? Be honest! Get feedback from others. Where, and with whom, are you trying to get your way by resisting, pushing, or manipulating? In what situations? What relationships? What are you trying to achieve by doing this? Which feelings might you be unaware of and/or avoiding beneath the surface? How is this affecting true connection with others?

2. Where might you be **passive**—letting things go, making excuses for someone else's behaviour? In what situations? What relationships? What are you trying to achieve by doing this? What might you be unaware of and/or avoiding? How is this affecting true connection with others?

3. Where might you be **passive aggressive**—pretending on the outside that things are fine, but acting aggressive or sabotaging behind the scenes? In what situations? Which relationships? What are you trying to achieve by doing this? What might you be unaware of and avoiding? How is this affecting true connection with others?

Next, review these next two questions and journal your thoughts and insights.

1. How might a lack of assertiveness be negatively impacting your life? How is it getting in the way of your health and wellness, your priorities and goals, or your dreams? Where is it getting in the way of true connections with others?

2. How has being non-assertive been serving you? (For example: *If I don't have these conversations, everyone thinks I'm easy going or a nice person. Or, if I behave aggressively, I can control the outcome and push people toward what I want. Or by unconsciously behaving passive aggressively, I don't have to take responsibility and face things (I can just blame others).*)

A Few More Pointers

Be real and be honest with yourself

This helps you *un* become as you move toward becoming. Becoming all that you really are may mean disappointing others, but it will mean becoming *you*. *Un* becoming means deprogramming the belief that we must keep the peace and not rock the boat, or that we must control others to be happy.

Assertiveness Is essential for Becoming You

Through my counselling and coaching practice, I've observed this struggle for many women over many years. So many women want to please. They don't want to disappoint. They want to be great employees, leaders, partners and Mothers. They don't want to complain, so they hold back. This results in being overwhelmed, and being drained—mentally, emotionally, physically, and spiritually. Sometimes, women who *are* assertive get *labeled* as aggressive. As women, let's support each other in our growth toward assertiveness. Don't call another woman aggressive or mean or controlling if she's been clear, direct, and respectful toward you or others. As women, we can support the *un* becoming for other women by encouraging these types of conversations, and by receiving feedback graciously. Support them when they have courageous conversations with you or others. Stop encouraging and expecting women, including yourself, to not set boundaries or say their truth when appropriate.

Assertiveness and Courageous Conversations at Work

You absolutely need assertiveness to deal with conflict at work. There are people from different family backgrounds, demographic groups, cultural groups and genders in one workplace. It's going to be complicated, and there will inevitably be disagreements and mis-understandings. There's nothing wrong with that, but how you deal with it matters. To you. And to them.

Not dealing with things is not an option because problems escalate, and negative feelings increase. Saying nothing is a passive form of aggression, and it will create more problems for everyone.

One of my clients shared how, when she approached her boss to discuss workload options for herself and her team, he became defensive and accusatory.

"You're always pushing," he said.

She wasn't pushing. She and her team were not able to keep up with the department's demands. There was confusion of roles among the team members, so some people were doing more, and some were doing less. She took some time to review what was going on before going back to her boss and explaining the negative impact being made by the lack of clarity.

He did not appear to like what she had to say. However, he realized that this was important, and he held a team meeting to clarify roles. My client was relieved. It was made clear who was responsible for what. As a result, some team members were in a bit of a disarray;

because my client and others had been picking-up a lot of slack, some people were suddenly faced with more work and responsibility, and they were not happy. This was a tough boundary for my client to set, but it was critical to sustaining her health and, ultimately, being successful in her work. She was brave to have this conversation with her boss.

I am enough and Self-Compassion

Being assertive and having courageous conversations is a way of showing yourself and others that you and they matter. It is a way of showing self value. It's how you build and strengthen your *I am enough* belief. Recognize and remind yourself that you matter. Your opinions, your beliefs, and your decisions all matter, and this is not based on what others think of you, but on what *you* think of you!

Questions for Reflection

As you consider the obstacles to courageous conversations, read over the following and choose one or two to reflect on and journal about.

1. How might your limiting belief(s) be getting in the way of courageous conversations?

2. Where might aggressiveness be showing up in your life and getting in the way of having respectful conversations?

3. Do you have a tendency to ignore your own feelings? Might this be getting in the way of courageous conversations? How so?

4. Do you have a tendency to give more than you receive in terms of time, money, and energy? What might you be getting from doing this?

Exercise: Review and Journal your Insights.

1. Write out areas of your life and relationships where you are assertive. Then, write about how this impacts you, others, your life, your wellness, etc.

2. Many women feel that by becoming assertive, they are giving up on being nice and compassionate toward others. What are your thoughts about this? Does it have to be all or nothing?

Courageous Conversations Case Study: Sally

Sally isn't sleeping well, and has been feeling exhausted lately. She wakes up late one morning and feels frantic about getting everything done so she can get to work on time. Instead of giving her kids a quick breakfast or asking her partner to help, she makes the usual breakfast, which takes more time than she really has. After all, that's what a good mother does. She grumbles and complains inwardly that her partner isn't helping. If he was paying attention, he would help. Why isn't he helping? She becomes more frustrated and resentful inwardly, but shoves this down.

She skips her own breakfast, throws on some clothes, and jumps in the car to head to work. As she is getting in the car, her cellphone rings; instead of ignoring it, she picks it up. It's her best friend Susan, who asks Sally to take care of her kids that evening while she goes to a yoga class. Overwhelmed, tired, and anxious, Sally says "yes, of course." She thinks to herself, "it's not that big a deal, Susan is just dropping her kids off at my house. And after all, helping a best friend is the right thing to do. It will be fine." She doesn't even notice her chest tighten, and the little knot in her stomach get stronger. Thoughts of 'why does Susan always ask 'me' to help' start to surface, but she quickly shoves those down, along with the resentment that is building. Sally rushes to work, still worried about being late. She can't be late. 'I have to be an exceptional employee' she says to herself.

'Sleeping in is never allowed'. Sally hates being late. It makes her look bad, and there's no excuse for it. "I just have a good work ethic' she says to herself. Late means irresponsible, and there's no way she is going to be irresponsible. As she says all of this in her mind, she pushes down her anxiety and overwhelm that threatens to bubble to the surface. And her chest tightens and her stomach starts to gurgle.

As she begins her workday, her boss appears and asks her to take care of something that is actually someone else's responsibility. That employee has not been reliable, so Sally has been picking up the slack. Quite a lot. After all, that's what good employees do. Although she feels resentful, she doesn't want to say anything or rock the boat. She doesn't want to look inadequate, irresponsible, or lazy. So, Sally says, "Sure, I can do that," even though she feels frustrated about it.

Resentment creeps up on her: why should she have to do this work, and why should she have to say something about it? Her boss should know that Sally shouldn't be doing someone else's work. Her mind becomes overwhelmed with these thoughts and her anxiety builds. But, she tries to push the resentment and negativity aside because she is scared of addressing her concerns. She doesn't want a conversation with her boss. So, as she tries to ignore them, her thoughts go back to her friend, Susan. She feels resentful toward her too, and then she feels bad about feeling resentful. Susan is a good friend. Why is she judging her friend? Sally goes back and forth between judging herself for feeling angry at Susan and being angry at Susan for asking her for help when Susan knows she's busy. Her thoughts go back to her spouse and how she feels she does everything for the family and that they can't even handle things if she sleeps in. Once! She becomes furious but talks herself out of saying anything to Susan, her boss, or her spouse because she decides that it's not that big of a deal. "I'll just let it go" she says to herself, because after all, that's what a good spouse, friend and employee do.

Can you relate to Sally?

The details may be different in your life, but you might be saying *yes,* when you need to say *no.* You may be tolerating something. You may not be having the conversations you need to be having to clarify boundaries or to say *no.* You are ignoring how you feel and what your body is telling you, and the resentment is building. Consider the areas of your life where you are tolerating things instead of having courageous conversations. What are you giving away? How much is it costing you?

What could Sally do?

She could start to see how people-pleasing or perfectionism is running her life. She could change her beliefs around this. She could determine her priorities, protect them, and say *no* to the rest. She could figure out what to let go of. She could ask her husband for help. She could say *"I'm sorry, but I can't"* to her friend. She could have had a courageous conversation with her boss about her workload. She could have paid attention to how she was feeling emotionally and physically—the resentment, the exhaustion, the poor sleep, the tightening in her chest, or the shallow breathing. But she didn't. Why? Her limiting beliefs kept her from taking care of herself and acknowledging, allowing, and accepting her feelings. Her need to please others or to be perfect overrode her need to take care of herself.

We all have days like Sally's. We all feel the weight of our familial, social, and professional obligations from time to time. The important thing is to keep working on our *un* becoming journey. With time, days like this will get less frequent because you will learn how to apply the tools you are learning from this book. Then, you'll be able to assertively communicate what you want and need in every aspect of your life.

When Courageous Conversations Don't Work—Difficult People

Courageous conversations are an excellent tool, but they don't work with everyone. For example, researchers estimate that one in twenty people has a personality disorder. I have studied this and worked for years with those impacted and people with personality disorders rarely change. They can, but it takes committed work and skilled therapy. I have counselled hundreds of people who have partners, parents, or bosses, who fall into the personality disorder category, and the only thing you can do when you are faced with this is to leave the situation when the behaviour is consistent and does not change. If you've had conversations and the other does not change. Stop.

Consider what water looks like when a stone is tossed in it. There are circles that flow out from the center. If you are close to the stone, the ripples hit you. The further you are away from the ripples, the calmer the water. The same is true with these types of relationships: if you are near a chaotic or problematic person, you will be impacted, regardless of how strong you are. You may need to set limits on people for a host of reasons, and you might need to adjust them over time. When a situation gets difficult, you may need to leave a person that does not show true remorse or a willingness to work on the behaviors they have that contribute to the problems in the relationship.

Even with all your best efforts, you will experience situations when others do not accept responsibility. They will avoid, minimize, ignore, deflect, change the subject, and blame you. At this point, you have a choice: ask yourself what you need and what's next.

- Do you need another courageous conversation?

- Do you need to set a boundary to protect yourself in some way? If so, what does that boundary look like? (Time away, a break or something else?)

- What is the level of the transgression and its impact on you? (Sometimes you don't really know this until you take a break from the individual).

- What are you willing to accept or not?

- What is the level of importance of the relationship?

- What is the level of your responsibility? As a parent or leader, whether it is at home or at work, you have a responsibility to hold people accountable. There may be consequences.

- Remember, it is not up to you to change the other person. It is up to you to have a conversation about the issue and then respond, perhaps by setting some boundaries and consequences.

Example: A close friend has been abrupt with you. As you reflect on the relationship you notice this has been going on for a long time. You recognize that this is really starting to bother you. You have the conversation, and they apologize, but their behaviour continues. What do you do? It is up to you. Do you feel that another conversation is warranted? Ask yourself again, is this what you want in a relationship? How important is this relationship to you? Do they have these patterns with others? This person may not value what is important to you. What are your next steps toward setting a boundary? A common confusion is believing asking for what we need is the only way to set a boundary. It's not. If we care about protecting our emotional, mental, spiritual and physical well being, saying "no" is necessary, but it may only be the first step.

The Second Step of Courageous Connections: Being Vulnerable

Real connection comes with vulnerability, and this brings the potential to deepen trust. When you share more, share deeper, share your insecurities and doubts, or share your dreams while someone else listens and acknowledges with support, you experience being accepted and understood. Being vulnerable takes courage.

Question for Reflection:

What would being more vulnerable and open look like for you? What relationship do you want to deepen in this manner? Consider who was in each of your circles. Reflect on the behaviors of this other person; do they listen to you? Do they show you value? Remember that those you are more vulnerable with need to have proven they will show up. That builds trust.

This requires courage, and it's one of the most powerful ways to *un* become. When others are *with* you and *hear* you, your willingness to explore your shadow increases. When everyone does the same, we help each other *un* become. When we bring more of what is hidden out into the presence of others, we heal. We can *un* become what is not us. It's safe and *un* becoming needs to be done within safe relationships.

The Third Step of Courageous Connection: Deep Listening

Real connection involves deep listening skills. The purpose of deep listening is to provide emotional safety so the other person to feels heard, understood, and thereby valued. This opens up the potential for deeper connection and provides the space for others to *un* become. People feel more connected to themselves when they're heard. If you have people in your life that you can connect to in this deeper way, consider how this feels to you, how valued and important it makes you feel, how it validates your own pain and human complexities, and how it makes you more deeply connected to yourself. Deep listening helps others go into their shadow by acknowledging their boulder. When we help others *un* become, it assists us with our boulders too. We aren't pushing another's boulder for them—instead, we're helping them see and accept their own boulder within the safety net of a powerful connection.

Un becoming can be a lonely process, but it is deepened when others hold space for us, and when we hold space for others.

The Important Components of Deep Listening:

- Acknowledge what they said with a thoughtful and compassionate response (e.g. *"sounds like this work situation is tough")*;

- Acknowledge how they feel with affirming statements (e.g. *"that could be discouraging")*;

- Ask questions to help them express themselves more deeply and show your interest and care for them. (e.g., *"how long has this been going on?" or "tell me more about this situation")*;

- Remember, listening is for *them*, not for you, and there should be no intention on your part to fix or change the other person.

Some of the Listening Mistakes that Impede Connection:

- We say things like: *"Yes, I have that problem too,"* and we bring the focus to ourselves, without any acknowledgement of them. We ignore them.

- We don't acknowledge what they said; we talk about something else, we are distracted by something we are doing, or we simply say nothing. We ignore them.

- We don't acknowledge how they feel. We ignore them.

- We don't inquire more to show that we care about them and their situation. We ignore them.

- We don't follow up with questions to help them go deeper. We ignore them.

- We are distracted, we don't look at them, or we are thinking about something else. We ignore them.

- We provide a solution or push for a particular approach to the problem. We tell them what we would do in that situation, what we've done in the past, or what we think they should do. We sometimes ask a question that implies a solution or something *you* think they should do, like, *"Have you forgiven that person?"* or *"What do you need to do to get past this?"* We ignore them.

- Our *why* questions are more about us than for them. We ask why because it doesn't make sense to us and it can come across as disputing and they may feel judged. Your deep listening is about them. Not you. We ignore them.

- We minimize their experience by saying, *"Oh it will be fine"* or, *"You can do it,"* or, *"Just be positive,"* without acknowledging how they feel first. We ignore them.

When we listen deeply, the other person has the opportunity to go deeper than they might on their own. Even conversations you may find trivial require deep acceptance if you want to truly show them support and deeply connect. If you can't listen to another person about superficial things, why would they trust you with deeper topics?

Acknowledgment

Empathy can be expressed by acknowledging someone's experience. You might say: *"That sounds hard,"* or *"It makes sense to feel that way."* This lets your conversation partner know that their experience is valid, and it opens up space for them to connect to (or acknowledge, allow, and accept) their own feelings. This is powerful. This can help them heal.

Sometimes, we offer advice instead because we are uncomfortable with someone else's pain, and we'd rather try to fix it for them. Doing this takes away their independence and their own ability to choose how to proceed. Be aware that when you do this, you may be doing it because you are uncomfortable with their experience. If people need advice, they will ask. Offering advice moves them out of feeling into thinking.

When we listen, we acknowledge and validate the feelings of the other person and, by doing, so we demonstrate deep understanding.

Trust grows when we really listen, and that's when connection happens. We need other people in our becoming and in our *un* becoming processes. Trust grows with the people who can be with us at our best and our worst. In that place, we are more likely to have the courage to face what gets in the way of becoming our true selves. This may be an invitation for you to be assertive and to ask others for what you need. You may need to ask them to listen to you in a way that honors you.

We all find ourselves on both sides of these conversations. It's in our awareness of what deep listening is that we can shift to provide this for those we love and care about. Know this: deep listening is one of the most powerful expressions of love for another.

Questions for Reflection on Deep Listening and Creating Connection

1. Review the facets of deep listening, acknowledging others' experiences and feelings, and then asking questions to understand and validate them. Think of a time when someone did this for you, and journal about the experience and what it felt like.

2. As you reflect on your deep listening skills, what might you do more of? Less of?

3. How might shifting to create deeper connections with deep listening help you on your journey to become *you*?

Summary

As this chapter comes to a close, here is a reminder: we discussed three ways to deepen connection with others:

- Courageous conversations are about clarity and respect. They are how you communicate your boundaries with the people in your life. Having these conversations helps you address what isn't you, and this helps you become who you really are.

- Being more vulnerable, sharing your failures, doubts, disappointments, deepest dreams, and desires with another person creates deeper connections.

- Deep listening is how you can hold space for another, build trust, and support someone else to *un* become.

Going Forward

Courageous connections require you to protect what is important to you.

Questions for Reflection:

1. Review your circle of relationships and consider what you want to enhance.

2. Given what you have learned in this chapter, what do you think might be the best way to achieve those goals?

    - A courageous conversation?

    - Being more vulnerable?

    - Listening more deeply? Or all three?

    - What are you ready to do?

3. What could be the potential gain for you and for the other person?

Going Forward: Questions for Reflection and Action.

1. How might developing the skill of courageous conversations help you in your personal life? Your work? How might it help the people in your life?

2. How might you want to stretch yourself with being more vulnerable and sharing more deeply with another?

3. How might you practice deepening your listening skills?

4. What will you commit to doing?

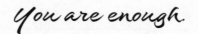

You are enough.

Chapter Nine

Managing Stress to Deepen Resilience

The Turning Point—The Power of *Un* Becoming to Becoming You

> "I am here for a purpose and that purpose is to grow into a
> mountain, not to shrink to a grain of sand. Henceforth will I
> apply ALL my efforts to become the highest mountain of all
> and I will strain my potential until it cries for mercy."
> —Author Unknown

Resilience is about putting together all the pieces we have covered to this point: self- compassion, recognizing and unravelling limiting beliefs, moving though emotions with intention and awareness, boundary setting, and courageous connections. You are beginning to notice how they all interrelate. You are at the fork in the road. You've been *un* becoming by attending to all of these pieces within you, and now as you *un* become, you are becoming who you really are. *Un* becoming *is* becoming.

In order to continue the process of *un* becoming, we need to be able to identify when life is too much and when stress is beginning to overwhelm us.

Sisyphus must have known and felt the stress. Pushing a boulder would be overwhelming in normal circumstance, let alone up a hill, continuously, with no rest, and never accomplishing his goal. How could Sisyphus have reduced his stress? He needed to notice, pause, and consider how he might do this differently. Maybe the heaviness of his boulder had to do with the fact that he was using old ways to try to create something new. It wasn't working. Pushing harder, working longer, and doing more, is not the way to move through stress. *As the saying goes, "The harder you push yourself, the harder your self pushes back."*

Not noticing is the first saboteur of resilience. Often, we don't even notice how over-stressed we are. We're just too distracted. In my training sessions,

I emphasize four things that are necessary to becoming more resilient and becoming *you*:

- Taking responsibility for our lives by noticing when stress becomes too much;

- Taking action by doing less or more of something;

- Addressing the underlying issues that drive your stress;

- Taking a holistic approach that addresses mind, spirit and body.

This book addresses underlying issues, helps you learn to take responsibility for your stress and what you are doing to make your boulder bigger. It also invites you to action, to do things differently.

We need to talk about stress. Building resilience requires that we understand what causes our stress. It requires us to understand how self-compassion, limiting beliefs, courageous conversations, and our ability to set boundaries and process emotions impact our stress levels.

Stress Management Assessment—Identify, Assess and Understand Causes of Stress

Take some time to assess where your current stress levels are and what may be the potential causes.

Come back to this checklist regularly as a way to assess and continue your awareness.

Answer based on how you are feeling presently:

1. **Symptoms of Stress.** Check all that apply:

    Physical:

    ☐ Tired

    ☐ Low energy

    ☐ Poor sleep (can't get to sleep easily, wake up through the night, wake up early and can't fall back to sleep)

    ☐ Over-eating

    ☐ Grinding or clenching teeth at night

    ☐ Migraines or headaches

    ☐ Tense muscles, shoulder pain, etc.

    ☐ Chronic aches and pains

    ☐ Sleeping too much

    ☐ Nightmares, bad dreams

    ☐ Exhaustion, shaking, nervousness

    ☐ Other:

Emotional:

- ☐ Anxious

- ☐ Overwhelmed

- ☐ Teary

- ☐ Sad

- ☐ Unmotivated

- ☐ Feeling apathetic, having trouble to get going

- ☐ Mood swings

- ☐ Excessive anger

- ☐ Irritable

- ☐ Feelings of emptiness

- ☐ Other:

Psychological:

- ☐ Avoid responsibilities

- ☐ Self-doubt

- ☐ Low self-esteem

- ☐ Negative thoughts toward self

- ☐ Negative attitude/thoughts toward others

- ☐ Lack of direction

- ☐ Indecisive

- ☐ Lack of hope

- ☐ Difficulty concentrating

□ Socially withdrawing

□ Excessive worrying

□ Catastrophizing

□ Excessive guilt

□ Other:

2. **Causes of Stress.** Check all that apply:

Work life:

□ Interpersonal conflict

□ Workload

□ Too much change, and it's happening too quickly

□ Emotionally draining work

□ Not enough challenge

□ Too much challenge

□ Lack of communication

□ Lack of clarification of roles and responsibilities

□ Job is not a good fit

□ Challenges with supervisor

□ Challenges with co-workers

□ Other:

Home/Personal life:

□ Lack of relaxation and/or recreation

□ Lack of exercise

☐ Lack of other self-care

☐ Too busy, doing too much

☐ Poor eating habits/poor nutrition

☐ Poor sleep

☐ Conflict with family and/or friends

☐ Financial concerns

☐ Health concerns, for self or others

☐ Other:

Self:

☐ Perfectionism—you push yourself too hard

☐ High expectations of self—you never feel like you're good enough, etc.

☐ Negative mindset/attitude toward self or others

☐ Over-analysis of challenges, other people, and/or yourself

☐ Victim mentality—"poor me" attitude

☐ Blame others for problems

☐ Over focus on situations or issues outside of yourself you cannot control

☐ Hold onto resentment; lack of forgiveness and letting go

☐ Do not acknowledge emotions to self; stuff and deny emotions

☐ Lack of assertiveness

☐ Poor choices:

  ☐ Poor boundaries (not saying no)

  ☐ Take on too much

  ☐ Put others first all the time

  ☐ Poor self-care

☐ People pleasing—giving in too easily, not setting boundaries

☐ Over-achieving—push self to do more, to succeed more

Now, take some time to reflect on your answers.

1. After completing this assessment, what do you notice?

2. What stands out to you?

3. How long have you been experiencing these symptoms?

As you read on, consider your answers and think about what you may want to do going forward.

How Does Stress Relate to Everything We've Seen So Far?

The following offers a review of all the material we've covered up to this point to help you see how all of the pieces interrelate and have the potential to help you become less stressed.

Recognize how self-compassion, understanding limiting beliefs, creating courageous connections, setting boundaries, and processing your emotions help you reduce stress.

Self-Compassion—Self-compassion reduces stress because it helps to increase your sense of self-worth. Through self-compassion, you are changing your beliefs about you. When you believe that you are valuable, you won't have to push yourself to be more and do more. You are enough. Self compassion also helps because there is less resistance to your feelings, an action which often creates more anxiety and stress.

Limiting Beliefs—It's helpful to realize which limiting beliefs hook you and when you're more susceptible to them. If you are more aware of when you are people-pleasing, over-achieving and being a perfectionist, you have more power to manage your thoughts, feelings and choices. Feeling empowered to deal with a situation will make it less stressful and changing the belief at the core of your over-doing will help you diminish stress. You'll be more empowered to set healthy boundaries.

Boundaries—When we set boundaries to manage our time and relationships, we are able to let go of what is not good or necessary in our lives. A huge cause of stress is simply doing too much or taking on responsibility for too much.

Emotions—Stress decreases for two reasons when we process our emotions:

- We are self-compassionate when we allow our emotions;

- We understand what is behind our feelings, so we have the power to make a better choice.

Questions for Reflection

Take your time. Journal your thoughts and insights.

1. How do you think the act of engaging in more self-compassion impacts your capacity to manage stress?

2. How do you think your increased awareness of your limiting beliefs impacts your capacity to manage stress?

3. What have you noticed about your stress level when you acknowledge and allow your emotions in a compassionate way?

4. What do you recognize about what you need based on how you feel?

5. How do you think that doing less and saying no affects your stress level?

6. How has setting boundaries reduced your stress? Journal any examples.

7. As you are becoming more aware of what creates deeper connections with others, what are you noticing about your stress?

Additional Tips to De-Stress

Small, Sustainable Steps or Practices
Create Long-Term Change

One of the most valuable lessons I have learned is that small, sustainable steps and practices create long-term change. You will not *become* overnight, however, as you take small steps, such as doing less, creating time for yourself, setting boundaries, engaging in daily self-care, or changing your thoughts, you will start to feel better and will build your resilience capacity.

Relax Regularly

Take time to slow down every single day, especially when life is more hectic.

Conscious Breathing

Being aware of your breathing is a powerful meditation all on its own. Find a quiet spot, close your eyes, and take some slow, deep breaths, inhaling and exhaling evenly for a few seconds. Research shows that pausing and taking just six deep breaths has tremendous health benefits, and it can help reduce stress. Follow your breath with your attention as it moves in and out of your body. Breathe into your body and feel your abdomen expanding and contracting slightly as you inhale and exhale. Notice how your breath feels on the back of your throat. Pay attention to your breath, imagine the oxygen, the fresh air you are breathing in, going into every cell of your body. Notice, even now, how your breathing has changed and your body is relaxing, as you read this.

Get Enough Sleep and Rest

Without consistent, restorative sleep, your cortisol levels rise, making it more difficult for you to fully rest and manage daily stressors. Cortisol also suppresses your immune system, making you more susceptible to flu, cold, and disease. Prolonged stress drives cortisol up, which can cause anxiety and other stress symptoms. Many people lose the ability to even know when their body is tired, let alone to know when they need a break. Check in with yourself and see if you are tired. Do this regularly. Rest is sacred, necessary, and essential to becoming who you really are. Rest honors the state of being. Doing, succeeding, attaining should not trump self care. I have come to see tiredness as a cue for me to slow down, shift inward, and learn to just be.

Our culture thrives on the glorification of a *strong work ethic*. This has become something we worship at all costs. It has a whole lot of unrealistic expectations attached to it, and they have nothing to do with being a good or successful person. To be successful we *hustle* so we work, strive, do more, give and give and wear ourselves out for the sake of something else. I have seen too many women allow their work ethic (which may be another word for perfectionism or over-achieving) worship trump their well-being.

This unrealistic expectation triggers our limiting beliefs, our need to be perfect, our desire to please, our tendency to over-achieve, and we continue to do more. It is another one of those instances in which we are trying to make ourselves feel better but actually end up feeling worse.

A few years ago, a friend of mine found herself exhausted, over-whelmed, disengaged from life, and losing interest in activities she had previously found pleasurable. She was in a job that was challenging and even inspiring at times, but she realized that it was holding her back. There was conflict among employees. There were roadblocks to her ideas. She was caught in a cycle of trying to fix everything, and she found herself carrying way too much responsibility. She usually arrived home exhausted, and she began drinking every day. She gained weight. She was not sleeping well, and she found herself obsessively reviewing details of conversations, thinking about what she said or what she should have done. She spent much of her time either working or ruminating about work. She hung on because she believed that she could change what was going on around her. To her, the idea of stopping or letting go of the responsibility for others felt like quitting, and she didn't want to be labeled that way.

Eventually, she did decide to leave her job. At first, she beat herself up over the decision, but over time, she chose to have the courage to listen to herself. Slowly, she made changes to her life. She changed her eating habits. She returned to her spiritual practices and explored new ones. She began to understand that she must take care of herself first. She realized that she had lived her entire life pushing herself hard, over-working, and only squeezing in time for herself. Eventually, she learned to make her own well-being a foundational priority. Even medical tests confirmed her physical healing. She was challenged by friends and family who were unable to accept her decision to leave her high-paying job with health benefits and a retirement plan. Having done this work on herself, she recognized what was most important was her embrace of her remarkable journey towards a healthier, happier, and freer life.

Manage Your Fears and Accept What Is

Fear is a primary cause of stress, anxiety, worry, and feeling overwhelmed. Fear of loss, fear of failure, fear of being hurt, fear of not measuring up, fear of not having enough time—all of it can contribute to physical, mental, and emotional stress. Fear of not being enough can keep our attention on the past or focused on the future, which adds to our stress. By completely accepting what is, you can let go mentally and stop resisting the issue or problem. Anxiety and stress may decrease, allowing you to relax.

Practice Being Positive

Research shows that a positive outlook on life can boost your immune system. Think about what you are grateful for and write it down. Practice thinking about five things you are grateful for each morning or evening before you fall asleep. What you think about as you fall asleep seeps into your subconscious and contributes to your reality. Think about what you do well and your positive attributes, characteristics, and accomplishments instead of focusing on what you are not able to do or what you lack. More about this in Chapter Eleven on Positive Psychology.

Get Connected

Find and maintain a supportive network of friends that suit your personality and your needs. Seek support when dealing with difficult events or challenges. Avoid or remove yourself from toxic and ongoing situations, including bad relationships at work and at home. Focus on connection and your boundaries.

How to manage stress more effectively—Summary

- Stop trying to do it all. Address limiting beliefs and negative self talk.

- Set priorities and be assertive.

- Ask for help and start saying no.

- Make better choices about your time. Do you really need to fill every moment with an activity?

- Process your emotions sooner rather than later.

- Practice being positive and grateful.

- Prioritize self-care.

Questions for Reflection

Consider one or two of the questions below and journal your thoughts and insights.

1. If you were to choose three areas or practices that are essential for your well-being, what would they be? (For me, it is enough sleep, daily brain practices, and time management.)

2. What are you presently doing that contributes to a sense of well-being and calm in your life? What will you keep doing?

3. What can you do in each of the following areas of your life to improve your overall health & wellness and reduce stress? Mentally, spiritually, physically. Reflect and write. Be aware it may not be reasonable to do them all at once. Consider focusing on one thing in each area.

4. If your stress is high right now, what is one thing you can do immediately to address this?

5. Consider all that you have been doing to take care of yourself these past several weeks or months. Write down what you've been doing in each of the following areas.

    · Self-Compassion

    · Limiting Beliefs

    · Creating Connections

    · Setting Boundaries

    · Emotions

    · Self-Care

6. What are you most proud of? Write down everything you've done to improve your life that you haven't written out yet. Be specific.

7. How does it feel as you reflect on all that you've done for *you*?

8. Which of your actions has had the biggest impact on shifting your life before the better?

9. How does all this create more capacity for you to *become* you?

Recognizing when we are stressed, and then doing something about, it is essential in maintaining and creating your well-being, which is an important facet of becoming who we really are. We can't be who we are if we allow over stress to remain.

Relaxation Technique: Practice Anytime.

The power to change happens when we do small things intentionally and repeatedly. There are many relaxation and meditations available. Here's an effective one you can practice for just a few minutes a day, either at work or at home:

1. Get yourself into a comfortable position and set the intention to take a few moments to relax and clear your mind.

2. Close your eyes and gently notice your breathing. As you attend to your breathing, you will notice how it slows down and softens. Notice and feel the breath on the back of your throat as you inhale. Notice and feel your breath as you exhale. Notice how you begin to relax.

3. When you're ready, think of a word that describes the way you want to feel (for example: peace, calm, love, or joy). On your next inhale, think of that emotion and how it feels and breathe it in. Imagine that feeling of peace or calm going into your mind, your heart, and every cell of your body.

4. As you exhale, imagine all the stress and worries leaving your body. You can even imagine that when you exhale, you are releasing toxins that disappear into the atmosphere.

5. Continue to do this as long as it feels good.

6. Each time you breathe in calm or peace (or whatever feeling you chose), imagine bringing this feeling in, starting with your head, then your face, then your arms, your hands, your fingers, etc. Extend the practice with your mind by breathing it into each part

of your body. Notice how your nervous system will become calm and be less over-activated.

7. Use this as one of your daily self care practices.

You are enough.

Section Three

Becoming *You*—Integration

More Support for Becoming *You*

Pain and hardship bring new growth. Our *un* becoming may be experienced as a form of suffering, in that we have the opportunity to dig deep and become who we really are. As in nature, new growth occurs after *un* becoming.

As you move into this section on becoming, you may notice that as you unravel what is not *you* and what has been getting in the way of you, you'll start to see yourself emerge. Much like physical health, when you remove what is not good for you (sugar, for example) your body and mind become healthier. You become more of who you really are by this removal. Addressing your limiting beliefs, the work you've done with boundaries, addressing relationships, and removing the things that are not you—can you see how in this *un* becoming you are becoming more *you*?

It might be a good time to pause and write down what you've done and what has changed for you, how you are feeling now, and how you have already become more of who you really are. Review your progress and how you've done it.

I know the work involved in *un* becoming, and I am proud of every step, every decision, and every choice you have made to get to this point. Big or small, each of these choices have honoured you.

You may be feeling that you haven't done enough, that you're not as far as you had hoped. I'm here to invite you to deepen your self-compassion once again. Remind yourself that you are enough. Always.

You may feel like you're *done*.

But here's the thing: there's more. These next chapters are gifts—they won't require as much effort as the previous ones. They will help anchor and deepen what you've already done, support you from slipping back, and help you get up when you do slip. Slipping back is not failure—it's actually an opportunity for progress.

The focus of this next chapter is your brain and how we can change it, thereby creating new health, new ways of being and feeling, and new ways of becoming more resilient and becoming the person you truly are

Chapter Ten

Brain Health & Nutrition

Your brain chemistry has a lot to do with your boulder. It might even be the physical cause of many of your struggles. When your brain chemistry is nurtured and healthy, it is much easier to become the real you—the you with more energy, focus, and joy.

The purpose of this chapter is to introduce you to the science of amino acid therapy and its impact on brain health. I am opening a door so you can get a glimpse into this science and start to grasp its potential life-changing impacts. I will help you understand the often-devastating symptoms of low brain chemistry and how you can determine if pursuing this avenue of therapy may be for you.

What does this have to do with becoming who you really are?

Brain nutrition addresses the physical cause of many of the emotional, psychological, and physical struggles that we face as women: low self-esteem, doubting ourselves, depression, anxiety, constant worry, insomnia, an over-active mind, excessive emotional sensitivity, over-planning, feeling overwhelmed, and even over eating. When we are able to address our nutrient-deficient brain with specific and targeted neuronutrients, many—if not all—of these symptoms are reduced, and even eliminated. When these are resolved, we are much more likely to become who we really are.

This chapter is only an introduction. I don't speak to the specific supplements that support brain chemistry and brain health, nor do I describe the details of the amino acid therapy protocol. That would require many more chapters, and there are already entire books written on the subject.

The protocol requires some mastery, and I will refer you to work by other experts, so you can more fully understand the process, set yourself up for success, and ensure your safety.

How I Found Amino Acid Therapy

I have engaged in this therapy myself and continue to do so, when needed. After working at this on my own and following guidelines in *The Mood Cure,* by Julia Ross, I went on to complete the Advanced Training and Certification in Neuronutrient Therapy. Following that, I earned a Master of Science in Health and Nutrition Education in order to be well-equipped to counsel my clients in this area. For my thesis, I researched and studied the impact of amino acid therapy on stress and reviewed several workplace changes for the women who participated. For both the Certification in Neuronutrient Therapy and my Master's of Science, I completed hundreds of hours of research on the topic of amino acid therapy and brain health.

Now, I have over fifteen years' experience in this area. In my work as a psychologist, I began to observe that in some cases, therapy was not enough to help my clients overcome depression or anxiety. They needed help with brain chemistry. Many of my clients responded well to this therapy and found that counselling or coaching flowed more smoothly once their brain was working better. As of the writing of this book, I am one of only a few trained in the world (and the only Canadian) trained by the NeuroNutrient Institute in Mill Valley, California, which teaches practitioners how to incorporate this information into their work.

Although this chapter introduces you to this protocol, I describe the next steps you can take if you'd like to read more on this and find a practitioner to work with, which I recommend. All of the information you need is outlined in the Appendix.

Finding the Missing Piece

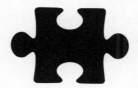

I refer to brain health nutrition as the missing piece to *becoming* because this area of science is neither widely known nor spoken about. In many cases, amino acid therapy can effectively address depression, anxiety, and more. All of the other information provided in this book is much more effective and easier to manage when one's brain is healthy.

As you *un* become, brain nutrition techniques like amino acid therapy, can help many of your stress symptoms, including poor sleep, anxiety, limited focus and concentration, and a busy, negative, cluttered mind. When your brain chemistry is addressed in this manner, you are more likely to have the ability to quiet your mind and, as a result, you are much more supported to become the real you. The boulder becomes lighter. There is less pushing against yourself and life.

You Are Not Alone

I experienced a radical shift in my life thanks to Amino Acid Therapy. Prior to implementing an amino acid therapy regime, I was functioning at a high level, yet still struggling. I had so little energy that even watching our kids' hockey games felt draining. Despite being so exhausted, I experienced insomnia. I felt apathetic and I had negative, and busy thoughts. I was also overweight, and I could not figure out the cause of any of it. When I sought medical support, the answers I received did not help.

The first weekend my husband and I started our amino acid therapy, we noticed an immediate shift. We were working together to renovate a room in our basement, and we both noticed that we were more lighthearted, less irritable, had more energy, and were even laughing and joking around. We completed the project together without getting on each other's nerves. This was a first! From there, we noticed that we had more energy after work.

I was not having to use my evenings and weekends to recover my energy, like I used to do. The constant tiredness and exhaustion started to lift. Other symptoms that I had not been aware of, like anxiety and worry, started to diminish too. My mornings weren't filled with as much worry and anxiety, and I was no longer waking up with that knot in my stomach. I started to sleep better, and for longer periods of time. I started to feel more rested. I was better able to focus on projects, and I wasn't getting as distracted or easily bored. Previously, I jumped from project to project and had difficulty staying on task. I recalled what Graduate School lectures were like--how hard it was to listen and absorb the information. After amino acid therapy, my mind became quiet and that continues to be the case most of the time. It changed my life and the life of many others—and the changes have been sustainable.

Given my career as a psychotherapist, and then as a Leadership and Brain Coach, I can attest to the increasing challenges many women are experiencing in the areas of depression, anxiety, and weight gain. High-functioning clients may not look like they are struggling, but they are. They are often fighting with their own mind, trying to quieten it, but to no avail. Some feel irritable much of the time. Executives and many leaders work long hours, and they have to think and make important decisions quickly that affect others. They are constantly synthesizing information, and they are under immense pressure to perform. My executive clients have reported many improvements with this therapy, which has greatly enhanced their own well-being and their ability to lead, communicate, and make decisions with more focus and calm. Many people view symptoms such as a busy, worried, unfocused mind, or feeling overwhelmed as a 'personality' trait. They've been this way for so long that they may think that it is simply who they are. But it may not be their personality. It may be their brain chemistry.

Without a healthy brain, relationships, work, personal life, setting boundaries, and assertiveness will be much more challenging. Amino acid therapy is the starting point with many of my coaching clients, particularly women, whether we are addressing leadership and executive competencies or personal development. True success, whether it is oriented towards leadership or one's personal life, starts with well being.

Exercise: The Four-Part Mood Type Questionnaire

(Used with Permission from Julia Ross), *The Mood Cure* by Julia Ross.

Rate your Symptoms: Put a number from 1 to 10 beside each symptom experienced, 1 "being slightly or hardly felt" and 10 being "strongly felt or felt all the time."

PART 1

____ Do you have a tendency to be negative, or to see the glass as half-empty rather than half-full? Do you have pessimistic thoughts?

____ Are you often worried and anxious?

____ Does your behaviour often get a bit (or a lot) obsessive? Is it hard for you to make transitions, to be flexible? Are you a perfectionist, a neat freak, or a control freak? A computer, TV, or work addict?

____ Do you feel guilty a lot?

____ Do you experience low self-esteem and/or consistent self-doubt?

____ Do you really dislike the dark weather or have a clear-cut fall/winter depression (SAD)?

____ Are you apt to be irritable, impatient, edgy, or angry?

____ Do you tend to be shy or fearful?

____ Do you get nervous or panicky about heights, flying, enclosed spaces, public performances, spiders, snakes, bridges, crowds, leaving the house, or anything else?

____ Have you had anxiety attacks or panic attacks (your heart races and/or its hard to breathe)?

____ Do you get PMS or menopausal moodiness (tears, anger, depression)?

____ Do you hate hot weather?

____ Are you a night owl or do you often find it hard to get to sleep, even though you want to?

____ Do you wake up in the night, have restless or light sleep, or wake up too early in the morning?

____ Do you routinely like to have sweet or starchy snacks, wine or marijuana in the afternoons, evening, or in the middle of the night (but not earlier in the day)?

____ Do you find relief from any of the above symptoms through exercise?

___ Have you had fibromyalgia (unexplained muscle pain) or TMJ (pain, tension and grinding associated with your jaw)?

___ Have you had suicidal thoughts or plans?

Refer to Chapter 3, page 25 in *The Mood Cure*. You may have Low Serotonin

Part 2

___ Do you often feel depressed—the flat, bored, apathetic kind of depression?

___ Are you often low on physical or mental energy? Do you often feel tired or have to push yourself to exercise?

___ Are your drive, enthusiasm, and motivation quotas on the low side?

___ Do you have difficulty focusing and/or concentrating?

___ Are you easily chilled? Do you have cold hands or feet?

___ Do you tend to put on weight too easily, or can't lose weight when you try?

___ Do you feel the need to get more alert and motivated by consuming a lot of coffee or other "uppers" like sugar, diet soda, ephedra, or cocaine?

Refer to Chapter 4, page 53 in *The Mood Cure*. You may have low catecholamines.

Part 3

____ Do you often feel overworked and pressured, or you feel the weight of deadlines?

____ Do you have trouble relaxing or loosening up?

____ Does your body tend to be stiff, uptight, tense?

____ Are you easily upset, frustrated, or snappy under stress?

____ Are you easily chilled? Do you have cold hands or feet?

____ Do you tend to put on weight too easily?

____ Do you often feel overwhelmed or as though you just can't get it all done?

____ Do you feel weak or shaky at times?

____ Are you sensitive to bright light, noise, or chemical fumes? Do you need to wear dark glasses a lot?

____ Do you feel significantly worse if you skip meals or go too long without eating?

____ Do you use tobacco, alcohol, food, or drugs to relax and calm down?

Refer to Chapter 5, page 77 in *The Mood Cure*. You may have low GABA.

Part 4

____ Do you consider yourself or do others consider you to be very sensitive? Does emotional pain, or perhaps physical pain, really get to you?

____ Do you tear up or cry easily—for instance, even during TV commercials?

_____ Do you tend to avoid dealing with painful issues?

_____ Do you find it hard to get over losses or get through grieving?

_____ Have you been through a great deal of physical or emotional pain?

_____ Do you crave pleasure, comfort, reward, enjoyment or numbing from treats like chocolate, bread, wine, romance novels, marijuana, tobacco or lattes?

Refer to Chapter 6, page 100 in *The Mood Cure.* These signs might point to low endorphins.

Now that you've completed the Four-Part Mood Type Questionnaire, read on to find out more about your symptoms, why you may have them and how you might address these.

The Four False Mood Types

Each section in the Four-Part Mood Type Questionnaire relates to specific brain chemicals: serotonin, catecholamines, GABA or endorphins. The symptoms of the four false mood types relate to each of these.

The Dark Cloud of Depression—Category 1—Serotonin

If you're high in serotonin, you'll be positive, confident, flexible, and easy-going. If you're sinking in serotonin, you'll tend to become negative (about other people and/or yourself), obsessive, worried, irritable, and sleepless.

Now, don't be confused by the title, "The Dark Cloud of Depression," because many of those who are serotonin depleted are not really down in the dumps or overwhelmed with sadness. Many are anxious, worn out, burned out, worry a lot, cannot turn their thoughts off, feel excessively hungry at the end of the day, want to eat more, or drink alcohol to calm down. According to Julia Ross's research, 50% of women are deficient in serotonin and experience varying degrees of the associated symptoms.

Results You May Experience with Plenty of Serotonin:

- Positive attitude.

- Emotional flexibility—being able to flow with change, conflict, etc.

- Sense of humor.

- Emotional stability—gets along well with others.

- Your mind will be more focused, less obsessive.

- Fewer carb cravings or cravings for drugs or alcohol.

- Improved sleep.

The Blahs—Category 2—Catecholamines

If you're high in catecholamines—which are dopamine, norepinephrine and adrenaline—you're energized, upbeat, and alert. If these have crashed, you sink into a flat, apathetic funk.

This is a different kind of depression (than the low serotonin depression), and it may leave you feeling unmotivated, low on energy, distracted, or unfocused. You may want to stay in bed all day or have trouble getting up in the morning. But you don't need to experience 'every' symptom to indicate low catecholamines. Even one symptom may indicate brain chemistry depletion and you could benefit from the therapy.

I find it interesting that when I ask my clients if they are depressed, most will respond that they are not. When we review the Four-Part Mood Type Questionnaire, most are experiencing symptoms in one or more of these four categories. I think this is because of education and what we have been told about depression. We have the idea that depression means that you experience very low moods, are very sad, cry a lot, and just feel, well, very depressed. Or we tell ourselves that we are not as bad as someone else, that in order to say that we are depressed, we must experience it severely. And yet, there are so many other symptoms that can indicate depression. Many of you are high-functioning. Despite how you feel, you still get stuff done! This sometimes makes us feel like we simply *couldn't* be depressed, because *real* depressed people can't get off the couch.

The other issue with saying that you are depressed is the stigma around it. So, I think it's important to say we have *symptoms* of depression, anxiety, or stress. Something else to consider along with the stigma is that we think it's our fault, so we don't like to admit it. We believe that we just need to do more or push harder. Pushing harder when you are depleted in the catecholamines can backfire and deplete your adrenals, eventually leading to adrenal fatigue. This can lead to serious chronic fatigue.

If you are low on these catecholamines, you may have such little *umph* to do anything, and, in fact, over-doing will further deplete any energy you have. It could plummet your brain chemicals even more. If you have symptoms in this category, you may also have low thyroid and require treatment for that. There's more detailed information on low thyroid and adrenal fatigue in the later chapters *of The Mood Cure*.

I also notice that many women find that they have to push themselves to be motivated and once they get going, they begin to feel more motivated and enthused, but it takes *pushing*, which is unsustainable in the long run. This *push* to do or exercise causes an increase in adrenaline, which floods the other neurotransmitters, thereby providing more energy and motivation. In the short term. This is not a healthy, safe, or effective way in the long run, and it may eventually lead to adrenal fatigue and exhaustion.

Results of Catecholamines:

- You'll be energized, upbeat, focused, and alert.

- More motivated and productive.

- Improved relationships—better ability to be focused and to listen.

Anxiety and Stress—Category 3—GABA

If you're high in GABA, you are relaxed and stress-free. When you're low in GABA, you may be wired, stressed, overwhelmed, feel constant pressure, have trouble relaxing, and your body could be uptight and tense.

Many women find that they are unable to cope with many regular day-to-day demands. Just *one more thing*, like the phone buzzing with a text or email coming in, pushes them to completely unravel. It's important to understand what is happening physiologically, or women will just blame themselves for not being able to handle it all. When there is continual stress over a period of time, your adrenals start to wear out, you get run down, and then even the small stressors can be too much for your mind and body to handle.

Many of the women I work with are chronically overwhelmed and stressed. Following this brain coaching approach, they find that they can handle challenging situations and relationships with more ease. They are more able to relax. Meditation, prayer, journaling and yoga become more effortless to engage in because the brain is quieter.

Results You May Experience When Your GABA Is Replenished:

- Calm and stress free.

- Better handle on stressful situations.

- Ability to manage more projects with ease.

- Less overwhelm.

- More able to relax and go with the flow.

- Less physical pain and tension.

Oversensitive Feelings—Category Four—Endorphins

If you're high in endorphins, you're full of cozy feelings of comfort and pleasure. If you're running out of endorphins, you'll be crying during commercials, feel overly sensitive, and get hurt easily. You may find it difficult to get over painful issues and losses, crave comfort food, and you may even experience more physical pain.

Those with low endorphins may be the sensitive people who take things to heart—although things may be going well for them, they are easily moved to tears. There is an emotional rawness in them.

How do endorphins get low in the first place? It may be that you have experienced more than normal emotional and/or physical pain. It may be because of stress or genetics. On average, women have lower endorphin levels than men do. People suffering from chronic physical pain have 60-90% less pain-reducing endorphins than others.

In my experience, one of the common symptoms that women with low endorphins may experience is over-sensitivity and/or crying easily. Emotional events seem to activate these sensitive ones more than others. Once the neuronutrients stabilize and endorphins are nourished, these women report feeling stronger. They can experience being with others in distress or pain without feeling overwhelmed by the other person's pain. The impact of this is enormous. Many say that they can receive criticism with less distress. They find that they can be present with others who may be struggling, without feeling overwhelmed emotionally or needing to withdraw or pull away. For those in the workplace who previously felt triggered or activated emotionally, they are elated to find that they can remain focused during these times. Receiving feedback is less stressful. They don't further deplete their energy by having to focus on holding in their emotions. They just simply are not overwhelmed by emotional pain like they once were. Imagine being able to allow your emotions without being overwhelmed by them.

High Endorphins Might Mean That You:

- Get pleasure out of life.

- Feel enjoyment *and*

- Contentment *and*

- Are able to recover more quickly from pain and loss.

- Are less sensitive to criticism.

- Are less emotional.

The Results

Once the neurotransmitters are addressed with the right neuro-nutrients (nutritional supplements including specific amino acids), we often see that depression, anxiety and stress decrease. Women sleep better. They have more energy. As you can expect, other things in their lives begin to change. If you are more relaxed, calm, and focused, you will lead with more awareness and mindfulness. You are more likely to be present and listen better. Relationships improve because your emotional reactions are more manageable. Science shows that addictions can effectively be addressed with this approach (see Joan Matthews Larson, PhD, *Depression Free Naturally* **and** *Seven Weeks to Sobriety)*. I started to notice that some women, including myself, experienced a deepening of their spiritual life following amino acid therapy. When the mind quiets, so much more is possible. Let's look at how these four areas of brain chemistry, when replenished with amino acid therapy, create change in the lives of women.

Addressing Low Serotonin to Feel Like Yourself Again.

A woman leader I was working with was ready to quit her job because she was so over-stressed and overwhelmed. She was a supervisor and, as a result of the workplace conflict, she was withdrawing into her office on a daily basis. She simply did not have the energy to deal with the conflict happening around her. She wasn't sleeping well, and most nights she slept on the couch in front of the television as an attempt to distract her mind so she could get some sleep. She was constantly tired and was gaining weight. She cried easily and was seriously doubting her abilities as a leader. Her confidence was taking a dive. Based on my recommendation, she started the amino acid therapy to address her low serotonin levels. Within two weeks, she noticed an astounding change—she was sleeping better and in her own bed, she was not feeling overwhelmed, her energy had increased, her depressive symptoms and anxiety had decreased, and she reported feeling like herself again. What she found so amazing was that her beliefs about herself had changed, too. The way she thought about herself was more positive, and she doubted herself less. She no longer ruminated about her mistakes. As a result, not only did she feel better, she was able to re-engage with her team at work. She had the energy and increased confidence to communicate and address the conflicts they faced.

Improved Catecholamines: Focus, Energy, and Mindful Leadership

One of my clients, an Executive, was curious about the amino acid therapy, not really believing she was experiencing any negative symptoms. She decided to complete the assessment, simply out of interest. Going through the questions helped her notice that her focus was not what she wanted it to be, and she recognized that her mind had a tendency to jump from one idea or thought to another. She had previously believed this was just her. Her personality. As a result, she was not as productive as she could be. She also had trouble focusing on what people were saying and really listening to them. She realized that she internally judged herself for constantly asking why she couldn't stay focused. Didn't she care?

During and following the amino acid therapy counselling, not only did her focus improve, she also experienced energy for a full day for the first time in years—no more afternoon slumps! Because she had learned to live with these slumps and accept them, she hadn't even noted them in her assessment. As her mind became more focused, she was able to be truly present with people in conversations and meetings, whereas previously, she struggled to focus on what people were saying, got easily bored, became irritated, often interrupted or checked out. Following her amino acid therapy, she felt calmer, more focused, motivated, and more energized. She was no longer fighting with her own mind. She was no longer pushing against herself. Could this perhaps assist with greater connection and the ability to deeply listen?

Improving GABA to Instill Calm.

GABA is a calming neurotransmitter. Many of my women clients are low in GABA and, as a result, are chronically stressed and overwhelmed, and find it very challenging to feel calm. One such client, with symptoms of low GABA, described her life as one stressor after another. She was having trouble sleeping and felt she needed wine every day after work. She shared that wine was the only thing that brought any sense of calm to her stressed body and mind. Once she started working with amino acids, she immediately felt calmer. The challenges at work and at home did not change, but her response to them did. She gave up her daily wine consumption. Not through sheer will-power—she just didn't crave it any longer. She was now providing her brain with nutritional support. She began to sleep better, and although she had not acknowledged that her body was stiff, tense, and sore prior to the therapy, she now shared that her body was feeling much more relaxed. The overwhelm and lack of calm she had been experiencing diminished greatly. Life had more ease for her. She also became more decisive and more focused on her priorities.

Improved Endorphins Lead to Balanced Emotional Responses

Many of my women clients describe themselves as overly emotional and find it challenging to not cry at inappropriate times. They may also feel deeply and find it hard to not take things personally. This was certainly the case for one client, whose deep feelings were causing her to over-identify with her employees and, as a result, found it challenging to remain objective and separate herself from their emotional struggles. She was over-empathizing with them and taking on too much responsibility for their struggles. This overwhelmed her and she became emotionally drained after conversations with them. Once she started the amino acid therapy to address low endorphins, we noticed a dramatic change. She looked lighter, happier, and stronger—but not hard. She still cared, and she was still strong. When she spoke, she was less teary. She was able to lead others and provide feedback, while separating herself from the responsibility to fix their problems. She was able to recognize others' responsibility for their behaviours. She said that she continued to empathize, but no longer felt emotionally drained by the conversations. This gave her more objectivity, a clearer mind, and she could stay present when speaking with others as opposed to trying to manage her emotional response. What a relief this was for her! She also found that her cravings for sweets and carbs diminished.

I had another client who completed an Emotional Intelligence Assessment prior to her amino acid therapy counselling with me. This was part of her leadership development. We then had her complete the same EQ Assessment *after* amino acid therapy, and the results showed a great deal of improvement in emotional awareness, managing emotions, and stress management. She felt much more stable and more comfortable with herself, and it showed on her second EQ Assessment. This was a direct result of the amino acid therapy.

Let's look at some other results: Here's a before, during, and after symptom comparison chart, tracking the change of just one of the hundreds of clients I have worked with over the past 15 years (where 10 indicates that she experienced that symptom strongly or much of the time, and 0 indicates that she did not experience that symptom at all). Notice the changes from June 9, at the start of the therapy, to September 20 of the same year, nearing the conclusion of amino acid therapy.

Jun 9	Jun 16	Jun 30	Sep 20	Symptoms of Low Serotonin:
7	7	7	2	afternoon or evening cravings
8	7	6	3	negativity, depression
10+	6	6	3	worry/anxiety
8	6	6	5	low self-esteem, guilt
10	10	8	3	obsessive thoughts or behaviours
10	9	7	2	irritability, rage
10	9	9	2	panic attacks; phobias; fear of heights, small spaces,
9	10	8	0	dislike hot weather
9	10	8	5	fibromyalgia, TMJ, headache (grind teeth)
9	9	9	2	night-owl, hard to get to sleep
8	7	5	2	insomnia, disturbed sleep

Jun 9	Jun 16	Jun 30	Sep 20	
10	8	7	4	nervous stomach, other GI problems

Jun9	Jun 16	Jun 30	Sep 20	Symptoms of Low Catecholamines:
10	8	3	2	apathetic depression
10	5	7	2	lack of energy
10	6	6	3	lack of drive, motivation
10	6	6	3	easily bored
10	7	7	4	lack of focus, concentration
10	8	6	4	ADD—like symptoms

Jun 9	Jun 16	Jun 30	Sep 20	Symptoms of Low GABA:
0	0	0	0	stiff, tense, painful muscles
10	8	8	3	over-stressed and burned out
10	7	5	3	unable to relax/ loosen up/sleep
10	8	8	5	often feel easily overwhelmed
10	9	9	0	hard to get to sleep

Let's review. You can see that many of her symptoms resolved, as indicated by a "0" near the end of her work with me. I chose this client as an example because although she was very resistant to the therapy and was very slow to engage in it, her symptoms improved remarkably once she embraced the process.

The difference for many of my clients is astounding. Many of the women I work with report more focus, which allows them to be more productive and present with others. They say that they are more patient with others and themselves. The harsh self-judgments and self-criticsm associated with people-pleasing, over-achieving, and perfectionism are lessened because negativity may result from low serotonin. Many women clients report an increase in confidence, a lessening of self-judgment, an ease in accepting themselves and being kinder and more generous toward themselves. In other words, they are more self-compassionate and more easily able to become who they really are. For one young mother, this meant being less irritable and more able to act like the parent she wanted to be. Many people are astounded at how quickly and effectively this works. They begin to notice other positive effects.

One young woman leader I am working with reported being able to plan and execute projects with less stress and worry, and with more focus. She says that she is less rigid and can let go of the over-organizing and over-planning that previously made her less productive and constantly occupied her mind. She reports improved communication with her husband. She is less emotionally triggered, and she is able to stay more mindful in potentially difficult conversations for a longer amount of time. Overall, many women experience less stress and an overall ease in their lives than they have ever experienced before.

Research Study—More Positive Results

Over a four-month period during my Master of Science degree, I researched and wrote a thesis on the impact of amino acid therapy on women. I worked closely with nine women who adopted the amino acid protocol. Over the course of the study, they made no other changes to reduce stress, no change in exercise, or even in their diet. (Although we typically address diet mid way in the therapy.) These results are based on self-reports, where the women rated each symptom prior to, and again following the therapy. I averaged the results and indicate it below as a percentage. Here are the results:

Results of My Study on the Impacts of Brain Coaching

All 14 stress symptoms improved: (Symptom listed first, then average % decrease of that symptom of the entire group.)

- Worry/anxiety—78% decrease

- Obsessive thoughts/behaviours—83% decrease

- Negative thinking—78% decrease

- Irritability/anger—86% decrease

- Panic attacks/phobias—100% (were eliminated)

- Controlling/rigid behaviours—40% decrease

- Poor sleep/insomnia—83% decrease

- Low energy—88% decrease

- Low motivation—50% decrease

- Poor focus/concentration—50% decrease

- Physical tension—71% decrease

- Stressed/burned out—63% decrease

- Overwhelmed—75% decrease

- Inability to relax—57% decrease

Workplace Changes:

Five of the women in my study went on to report the following workplace changes following four months of amino acid therapy. At the end of 4 months, the following 8 workplace competencies (that were assessed) improved:

- Almost 40% average improvement in engagement, assertiveness and emotional self-management.

- Productivity—22% average improvement

- Relationship with boss—30% average improvement

- Performance anxiety—32% average improvement

- Conflict management skills—36% average improvement

These results demonstrate the potential impact of amino acid therapy. The proper regimen can improve your personal, social, professional, psychological, spiritual, and physical well-being.

How Amino Acid Therapy Assists with *Becoming*

High or Abundant Serotonin

When you're high or abundant in serotonin, it will be easier to be more self compassionate and less critical of yourself and others. Your mind will be quieter, and you'll have more confidence. You will ruminate and second-guess yourself less. Your need to people-please, be perfect or over-achieve may be related to obsessiveness, which is related to low serotonin. As you feel calmer, you may be able to set boundaries and have conversations with less worry and anxiety. When others provide you with feedback, you may be able to take it in more easily. You may find it easier to get restorative sleep, as low serotonin is one of the culprits for insomnia. Serotonin also provides courage, so having courageous conversations may be easier for you. Self-care, such as eating healthier and drinking less, may occur because addressing low serotonin levels helps diminish cravings in these areas.

High or Abundant Catecholamines

You'll have more energy for self-care routines, such as exercise, or shopping for and creating healthy meals. Your mind won't jump around as much, so your ability to deeply listen will be improved, and it will be easier to create deeper connections. You'll have more "umph" for work and daily activities, and you won't get depleted as easily. You may not have the need to be as busy, so you may be able to slow down and honor yourself in new ways. Being easily bored is one of the symptoms of low catecholamines. This keeps women focused on doing and being busy, which as we know, can diminish wellness, connection to self and others.

High or abundant GABA

Overall, you'll be less stressed. If you're less stressed and overwhelmed, it may be easier to connect with others, be less critical of yourself, and be able to go with the flow. As a result, it may also be easier to make better choices and set boundaries for yourself. You'll have an increased ability to stop and reflect on the choices you want to make on your journey toward *becoming*. You may sleep better, too.

High or Abundant Endorphins

With less emotional pain, you may not feel as strong a need to fix others' struggles. You may be less people-pleasing and be able to have courageous conversations more easily because you don't become overwhelmed with emotion. You may be more self-compassionate, and you may experience diminished drug, alcohol, and carb cravings.

What if the next step—or even the first step—in your self-care journey, was amino acid therapy? If you are interested in finding out the exact nutrients that support this process, the resources and books that explain this in detail can be found in the Appendix at the end of this book.

Other Ways to Support your Brain Chemistry

1. Protein. Eat three meals a day with sufficient protein at each meal. Protein is necessary to support your brain chemistry and therefore, healthy moods.

2. Healthy Fats, like omega 3 oils, feed the brain. Eat healthy fats like butter, olive oil, and avocados are a great start.

3. Avoid these foods: sugar, white flour, and caffeine. They deplete your brain chemistry and do not support good health.

4. Create simplicity with your food intake. Whole foods, preferably organic, as well as high quality protein, plenty of fruits and vegetables, and lots of filtered water.

Questions for Reflection

Choose 2-3 questions and reflect on and write out your responses.

1. Now that you have read this chapter and completed the brain chemistry assessment, what area of brain chemistry might be the most depleted for you? How might this be affecting your health, your life?

2. Which of my clients' stories did you relate to? How so?

3. What might be the benefits or potential impacts for you, if you do address neurotransmitter deficiencies with this nutritional approach?

4. Write down the three main symptoms you are experiencing that could potentially be related to a depletion in brain chemistry. Refer to the assessment at the beginning of this chapter. Can you find an alternative explanation for those symptoms?

5. How might addressing your health and wellness in this manner be a way of exercising self-compassion? Self-care?

6. What might be your first step in addressing this depletion?

7. How might this way of tuning into yourself support your growth and development in other areas of your life?

In my experience, those who embark on this approach find that in order to be successful, they need to tune into and pay attention to themselves, their body, their mind, their emotions, and their spirit at higher levels. This is a way to support their self-care practice and self-compassion, helping them to *un* become what is not them and become who they really are in a powerful way.

Going Forward

- Consider how brain health therapy may support your self care.

- If you want to pursue further assistance in this area, the resources, and where to find a practitioner is listed in the Appendix. I am a trained practitioner, so you can also always reach out to me.

- Continue to focus on just one area of *becoming you* practices and continue to practice new ways of being and acting in each of these areas. Those areas may be strengthening your self-compassion, addressing limiting beliefs, working on boundaries, having courageous conversations, or practicing being with your emotions. Just focus on one.

- Review what you've been doing well. Take time to reflect on all of your achievements on the way to becoming who you really are.

You are enough.

Chapter Eleven

Positive Psychology and Neuroscience

"90% of long-term happiness is predicted not by the external circumstances but by the way your brain processes those events."
—Shawn Achor research study, 2013

If you want to boost your mood, become more resilient—even happy—and not be pulled into downward negative spirals, then you'll want to explore the life changing power of neuroscience and how to practically apply it to your life. Positive psychology and neuroscience techniques have the power to change your brain, how you view yourself, thereby changing how you feel, and consequently changing how you live your life. The techniques I share in this chapter will assist you in becoming more of who you really are, through letting go and minimizing the negativity in your mind. These techniques will support the other work you've been doing in *un* becoming what wasn't you. By engaging in these techniques, you create a base of positivity vs. negativity in your mind that will allow you to handle the stressors of life with greater ease, including your *un* becoming.

What is Positive Psychology?

Positive psychology looks at what is right with you and with others and situations. It is not an avoidance of challenges or negative emotions, but rather focuses more on what could be—ways to flourish and expand as opposed to what isn't working.

Research shows that when people have a positive mindset, their performance on almost every level, including productivity and creativity, improves. Imagine what is possible when we learn how to remain in a more positive state of mind!

What does this have to do with becoming who you really are? When we consider who we really are and becoming that *real* us, positive psychology and neuroscience techniques can provide enormous support. This work can change or lessen our negative thoughts and beliefs about ourselves, lessen the intensity of our emotional responses, and help clear the way for us to become who we really are. Our mind is clearer and more positive, and we are more able to live our lives with more ease and less stress and overwhelm.

Positive psychology for women is good news. As I've mentioned, women tend to be worriers, we struggle with self doubt and we tend to think negatively of ourselves—thus the *I'm not enough*. Since, as women, we have this negativity bias and tend to overthink and ruminate as a result, the information and techniques I provide here will be very helpful in becoming who you really are—a more calm, joyful, and motivated woman.

The Positive Brain

So, what is actually happening in the brain when we focus on the good? The science of neuroplasticity actually means that the brain can be changed. This means that when we direct our thoughts from the negative and toward the positive, we create new neuropathways. In *You Are the Placebo: Making Your Mind Matter,* Dr. Joe Dipsenza writes: "Self directed neuroplasticity (or SDN) means we can direct the formation of new neural pathways and the destruction of old ones through the quality of the experiences we cultivate." In other words, simple practices or micro habits, where we regularly focus on or imagine the good, have the potential to create new neuropathways and diminish the old, destructive ones.

The negativity bias is basically our pull to see, notice, and stay with what's wrong in a situation. We may be feeling fine one moment, but an event, comment, or piece of bad news pulls us to notice and focus on the worst aspects of a situation. Many women fall into the habit of reminding ourselves of our failures, telling ourselves we are not enough or that we are worthless, and so-on. It takes intentional effort to undo this, but it is possible.

Dr. Rick Hanson, the author of *Hardwiring Happiness,* suggests that this bias creates two problems:

> *First, it increases the negative. It pulls your attention to what is or could be bad, makes you overreact to it, and stores the negative experience in implicit memory. [...] This bias increases your stress, worries, frustrations, irritations, hurts, sorrows, feelings of falling short, and conflicts with others. Second, the negativity bias decreases the positive. It slides your attention past the good facts around you. It makes you underreact to the good facts you do notice.*

What was going through Sisyphus's mind as he pushed that big rock up that big hill? Did he tell himself that he deserved this punishment? Did he complain that this was someone else's fault? Did he moan, 'This will never change, I will never get to the top?' Did he curse the rock? We could imagine a million negative thoughts that may have endlessly raced through his mind. As you have worked through the concepts in this book, you are likely becoming more aware of your self-talk, that inner voice that reminds you of your failures, that you're not enough, or that you don't do enough. Although you are more aware of your critical inner voice, it can be challenging to shift it. Self-compassion, as discussed, is one of the ways that you begin to change your negativity toward yourself. The practice of positivity is another way.

Repeatedly practicing positive experiences and feeling the emotions that coincide will help pull you out of this negativity bias. You'll become more resilient and much more equipped to handle challenging events and life circumstances that could otherwise sidetrack you. The purpose is to help you more quickly experience a place of peace and contentment, regardless of what is going on around you and in your life. You're more able to manage your inner critic (e.g. *you're not enough, you have to be perfect, you have to please everyone, you have to do more*) and diminish its power over you. This does not diminish the need to accept what you are feeling without judgment. It simply trains your brain to not go down the rabbit hole of despair, anger, hurt, or frustration every time or for as long. With the power of practical brain exercises (neuroscience) you will provide immeasurable support to yourself as you become the real you. Essentially, these brain exercises assist you in *un* becoming what is not really you. You will be able to be more objective about situations and your emotions won't be as overwhelming. You will complain less. You will focus less on the negative aspects of other people as well as yourself. It is not the positive event, or the situation you are imagining that creates change in your brain, it is the emotion. Positive emotions change the brain.

The "Big Three"

One of my clients who struggled with the belief that she was not enough took on a series of exercises that dramatically shifted her mindset and, consequently, her life.

When I first met her, she felt very anxious. In order to manage her anxiety, she micro-managed others and engaged in other behaviours that diminished her power as a leader. In her personal life, she was feeling very over-stressed and, instead of slowing down, she pushed herself harder. She agreed to practice the following three simple micro habits daily:

1. Choose a feeling word or intention for the day and meditate on this.

2. Flip your belief by thinking of something you struggle with and say the opposite to yourself. Notice how you feel.

3. Review of your day. What was good about this day? (Many of you have experienced the power of gratitude, and science supports how gratitude changes the brain.)

These micro habits resulted in a major decrease in stress and anxiety for my client. She showed up to presentations in a whole new way. She slowed down her speech. She asked questions, which she hadn't done before—she had believed that, as the leader, she should have all the answers. She paused. Ultimately, she began to trust herself more, and she was able to let go of her negative self talk.

I also suggested that she review her successes from time to time and ask herself what she did well. This was intended to further anchor the positive changes in her brain. As a result of these brain practices, she was gradually able to lessen the need to be perfect and please everyone. She had lessened her boulder, and she was becoming more herself.

Exercise—The Big Three

1. **Five minutes in the morning**

   Practice saying just one feeling word for the day for a minimum of four days. Set your intention each morning to feel love, peace, calm, or joy (or something else). You get to choose what you want to feel. Imagine an experience (real or imagined) which makes you feel good. Visualize that experience and imagine what it feels like. Pay attention to the positive emotion. Pause with the emotion. Take your time with this. Feel it in your body by imagining the feeling deep in every cell. You can come back to this feeling any time, when you are driving to work, driving home from work, working, eating your lunch, doing a task, or more. After four days, reflect on any changes. What are you noticing within yourself? Continue to do this daily.

   Your brain cannot tell the difference between what is real and what is not, so *imagining* a positive experience feels real to your brain. This is the power of your mind in creating pleasant and positive feelings and experiences. You are essentially creating micro habits of these daily exercises. There is much that happens in the body and brain when you deepen the positive experience by feeling it. Serotonin and endorphins, your feel-good brain chemicals, are released which impact the way you feel in a positive way. You also begin to calm your limbic system, which over time, unaddressed, can cause you to overreact to every perceived threat due to life's hardships and challenges. Your brain can get in the habit of making you feel worse, so the opposite is true as well. You can get your brain into the habit of making you feel peaceful, calm, upbeat and happy.

2. **Practice flipping your belief**

   This exercise, which was developed by Pam Grout in her book *E-Cubed*, involves re-framing negative thoughts about yourself.

Throughout the day, for the next four days, think of something you struggle with and begin to say the opposite to yourself as often as you remember to. (This term and concept, *flip your belief* was coined and explained by Pam Grout in her book, *E-Squared.*) For example, if you struggle with low confidence, repeat to yourself: *I am confident.* Then, notice the evidence of this new statement. After four days of adding this to your daily routine, journal what you are noticing. When happier thoughts occur and you think them repeatedly, new synapses form and strengthen, making it easier to access happiness when you need to. This type of *flip your belief* practice affects the prefrontal cortex, which is the part of the brain that manages emotions and behaviours. Because we are talking about becoming who you really are, you will also discover, through practices like this, that your focus, motivation, and creativity improve—all of these are functions of the prefrontal cortex.

3. **Review of your day**

After you have engaged in the first two practices for about a week, begin to add this third practice to the end of your day. Before you go to sleep or as you lay your head on your pillow, review what was good about your day. Do it slowly, reflecting on each good thing. Some start with writing these good things down in a journal. These thoughts will produce positive emotions, and you will fall asleep thinking about the good rather than reviewing what didn't go well about your day. Fall asleep thinking about the good and allow the positive feelings to deepen into your subconscious. You are taking charge of your thoughts instead of allowing them to run rampant. You are reviewing what you didn't get done, what you did poorly, what you need to do the next day, who didn't measure up or how you didn't measure up, and on and on. As demonstrated by the work of Dr. Richard Davidson, professor of psychology at the University of Wisconsin, the left prefrontal cortex is more active when people feel happy. So, what stimulates the left prefrontal cortex? Repeated exposure to positive or pleasant thoughts. Think positive and you can change your brain.

What We Focus on Grows

Another woman leader I was coaching started to practice only the *flip your belief* exercise. She greatly undervalued her contributions to her organization and found herself caught in a cycle of declining confidence. Given this cycle of low confidence that she had created, she chose to tell herself that she was confident. I told her that she didn't even need to *believe* she was confident right away—she just needed to say to herself, *I am confident,* consistently. So, she did. Throughout the day, she would flip her belief to *I am confident.*

The other component of this process is to notice the evidence of this new belief, as I have mentioned. This client began to notice as she flipped her belief, she felt calmer; she noticed and reflected on this. She began to notice when she felt calm, her thoughts were clearer, allowing her to communicate with more ease and clarity. As she noticed these changes, this allowed for genuine confidence to grow. This was the evidence she needed. She looked for more evidence and, over time, she began to believe that she could do the job. Her confidence improved even more. The key was flipping the belief daily, and then noticing the evidence of this new belief as it started to materialize.

When she felt herself slipping (and the old *I can't* or *I am not enough* thoughts started coming back), she focused on what she had accomplished, not what she didn't get done. This actually gave her more energy and motivation, and she found herself not only happier, but more productive. The brain defaults to the negative. We need to *train* it to focus on the positive. She did this with *one small practice.* This created *huge* change for her, and it was a catalyst for many more positive changes in her life.

A few years ago, I took it upon myself to practice just the *5 minutes in the morning* intention exercise of the Big Three. After about two weeks, I noticed some remarkable changes:

- Prior to this practice, I was anxious and could feel it in the pit of my stomach when I woke up every morning. If I wasn't anxious, I felt rather ho-hum and *blah*. As I focused on my positive intent (by choosing to feel peace), I noticed that I could shift my mental and emotional state. Sometimes the feeling of peace came immediately, and sometimes it took some time. It was working. I was able to *choose* to feel this feeling.

- I noticed that when I thought of life's worries, I was more quickly able to shift out of it and feel peace again. When I noticed, I could choose to stop thinking about something and choose to start thinking about something else, without an enormous struggle.

- I found that I complained and vented less, and when I did, I didn't do so for as long.

As Norman Doidge, MD, explains, in his acclaimed book, *The Brain that Changes Itself: Stories of Personal Triumph from the Frontiers of Brain Science*:

> The brain has the capacity to rewire itself and form new neural pathways—if we do the work. Just like exercise, the work requires repetition and activity to reinforce new learning.

If you think about it, you are always talking to yourself or thinking about something. If you are allowing a constant barrage of *I'm not enough*, *I can't do this*, or *I'm not capable enough* beliefs, you will feel anxious. This anxiety is partially a symptom of an overstimulated amygdala (the emotional centre of your brain) which can be caused by *your* negative thinking. When you start to notice your thoughts and shift them to more positive ones, your amygdala will start to feel less stress, and so will you.

Overcoming Fatigue and Overwhelming Feelings

One of my clients, Theresa, was worn out, feeling discouraged, and did not have the zest for life she once had. She started to *un* become through this daily practice of reviewing her day in a positive manner, but she felt that something was still missing. Then, Theresa started doing one thing. She started sitting for fifteen uninterrupted minutes in the evenings and reviewed what was good about her day. Sometimes, she would enjoy a cup of tea. Sometimes, she journaled the good things and other times, she simply sat and reflected on what was good. Alone. At first, she only considered the *big stuff* as good, like getting a great performance review at work, or having lost weight, or paying off her mortgage. But as she continued this practice, she trained her mind to see the good in almost every circumstance— noticing a flower blooming, noticing a colleague who thanked her, noticing that gas prices went down two cents, or noticing her children's kindness. What transpired was truly remarkable. She looked brighter, she had more energy to spend with her children, she was more patient with them and herself, and her zest for life returned, both at work and at home. She too was pleasantly surprised how this one seemingly insignificant practice changed how she felt.

Sound too easy or simplistic to be effective? The smallest things are the biggest things. In other words, the regular practices of small changes like one or all of The Big Three can produce remarkable change.

Reflections on Self-Compassion and Brain Practices

Self-compassion, or simply being kind to yourself, helps build these same resources in your brain. These brain practices are self-compassionate—they are self-care in action.

- Review your day as you drive home and talk to yourself like you would a friend, not just when times are tough, but any time.

- Encourage yourself! We provide enormous encouragement to others when we tell them they've done well or done great work. Doesn't it make sense to be our own biggest supporter?

- As you drive to and from work, engaging in errands, or go for a walk, take in the good. Notice the trees, the sky, the children playing in a park, and take it in the good feeling. When you go for a walk, practice intentionally noticing nature around you: the trees, the flowers, the grass, the water. Take it in. Deepen the good feeling.

Gratitude and the Brain

A study conducted by Prathik Kini out of Indiana University recruited 43 participants. The participants had self-identified as suffering from anxiety and/or depression. Half of the group was assigned a gratitude exercise that consisted of writing letters of thanks to various people in their lives. The other half did not engage in this exercise. Three months later, all 43 participants had brain scans.

Kini found that "the participants who'd completed the gratitude task months earlier not only reported feeling more grateful two weeks after the task than the control group, but also months later, showed gratitude-related brain activity in the scanner. The researchers described these 'profound' and 'long-lasting' neural effects as 'particularly noteworthy." (Christian Jarrett, Science of Us blog)

Studies like this show us that our brains can change by focusing on the good. Gratitude and positivity can calm the limbic centers of your brain and not only make you feel better and more optimistic, but also strengthen the decision making center of your brain, thereby making you more focused and motivated to complete tasks and goals.

Dr. Danie Amen, a world-renowned neuropsychiatrist and brain scan expert, conducted a *before* and *after* brain scan for a psychologist who was writing a book on gratitude. The first brain scan took place after she had meditated for 30 minutes on what she was thankful for. The brain scan showed her brain looking healthy. Days later, the psychologist focused on her major fears for a time. The following brain scan indicated decreased activity in her cerebellum and temporal lobes. These areas are responsible for cognitive functioning and coordination, which could indicate why we have trouble processing information and are sometimes clumsy when under stress.

Exercise

Read through the following and choose one or two suggestions to reflect and journal on. These will help you anchor good feelings into your brain an create new neuropathways:

1. **Review your past week.** Think about some of the work you accomplished, your conversations, and your interactions with others. What did you do well? For example, *I was patient and kind to the store clerk. I offered some extra time to one of my co-workers. I drank more water. I exercised for 3 days. I offered some great ideas in the meeting yesterday.* Try to say it in the positive by thinking things like *I was positive and encouraging* rather than *I was less irritable or less angry.*

2. **Review one of your goals and encourage yourself**. It may be something like *I've done well setting boundaries,* or *I said no to this, I said no to that.* You will become your own biggest source of encouragement, and you will feel better, more energized, and more motivated.

3. **Write out the Big Three steps on a small card.** Decorate it, doodle on it, laminate it, and keep it with you to remind you of these micro habits. These could be your three self-care practices for each day.

4. **Keep it positive.** Write out what you are grateful for, reflect on your vision board, or create one now. Review and reflect on what you wrote for the vision of your life in the Introduction and reconsider what your life would look like if everything was going as well as possible.

5. **Pay it forward.** Acknowledge positive characteristics in other people by thanking them and being specific about the positive things you see in them. For example, you could tell someone, *you always seem to see the good in people* or *you are always so grateful when I offer you something.*

Regardless of the positive impact these brain exercises have, everyone slips occasionally. Know that it is normal. It has been my own experience. The brain sometimes resists our best intentions, especially as we are working to rewire it.

When to Feel Emotions and When to Flip the Belief

Always acknowledge what you feel, even if it feels like an exaggeration. Acknowledge and allow the feeling. From here, you can flip the belief and say the truth to yourself. This can be part of the reframing stage that I shared about in Chapter Five on Emotions. By doing so, the intensity of your emotions may subside—perhaps not always, but more often. This is also a way of showing compassion to yourself.

A criticism of positive psychology is that it may be overused and diminish the acknowledgment and awareness of life's challenges as well as genuine human suffering. As I see it, these practices help to cushion intense feelings, but not with the intent of ignoring them.

Many find that the feelings subside more easily with this work because the negativity gains less traction. It's like exercise: the daily practice of physical activity increases one's well-being and can help prevent injury, but that doesn't make it a good idea to ignore the pain that tells us we have an injury.

These brain practices make you more resilient to negativity and unhappiness, and they help you cope through those difficult times with more ease. Saying *oh you'll be fine, just think positive thoughts* to yourself or when someone is struggling is a misuse of positivity.

Summary

- Positivity can change your brain and shift you out of negativity more quickly.

- These daily practices help to create physiological change in your brain. The smallest things can create the biggest change.

- You can practice positivity any time and place. Remember, it is the positive feeling that creates the biggest and most lasting impact.

- This is important for women, as this can improve our confidence, reduce our worry and self doubt, and help minimize the anxiety and overwhelm many of us experience.

Questions and Reflection

Practice one or more of The Big Three for four days, then answer the following:

1. Which of The Big Three brain exercises do you feel drawn to? What might work for you? What might you start doing? Continue doing?

2. If you have been trying out any of these exercises, what have you noticed? Journal what is improving or changing even slightly.

   a. Is there anything else that you can do to implement 'The Big Three' into your life on a daily basis? Consider setting up a reminder to pause throughout the day and practice one of The Big Three exercises.

   b. Reflect regularly about how this is helping you. Discuss within your group of women (if you are meeting with a group) or find another way to keep yourself accountable to your practice.

3. Consider using The Big Three as your daily self-care practices.

4. As you reflect on where you are, how might the information and practical suggestions in this chapter support you as you become more of who you really are?

You are enough.

Chapter Twelve

Creativity & Spirituality—Connecting Within to Become More *You*

*"The spiritual life does not remove us from
the world but leads us deeper into it."*
Henri J.M. Nouwen

From me to you:

*Sometimes, I wonder how I can be pulled outward as I desire
to go inward. Sometimes, my worlds feel at odds, and I believe
that somehow, reconciling it is important. I am very drawn
to the inner-world of my being, so I slow down, and although
peace emerges, I feel pulled to the outer world of my doing.
It's in those moments that I remember that I am both.*

Spirituality Has Been Here All Along

The invitation to explore our spiritual lives requires an awareness of the integration of all that I have shared so far. Setting

boundaries and having courageous conversations, slowing down and facing what is painful, letting go, becoming more self-compassionate—all of this helps to integrate you and your true essence. On its own, all of this is simply information. When we integrate these concepts, take the time to reflect on how they transform us, and begin to 'act' differently, we enter the spiritual realm—the place of mind-heart connection— and we become more of who we really are.

This is important for women because if we ignore our heart, we lose connection with ourselves. Spirituality provides a holding space for women to become their real selves, integrating the knowledge and understanding we need within our true selves. Much of this book has been about how society and us pull us from ourselves, as women, causing us to live by *pushing* rather than by *being*.

Spirituality is an invitation to you, to integrate all of who you are and settle into your being ness.

Spirituality is also a brain practice. Allowing your brain to work as a whole means connecting your emotions, thoughts, beliefs, creativity, and intuition. By doing so, you also connect to a higher self, or what some people call a higher power.

When we pray or meditate, our brain waves change. They slow down and enter an *alpha brain wave* state, which is important because it allows two things to happen:

- We have more direct access to our Higher Self/God/ The Creator/Consciousness;

- We can create more change in this state because we have more direct access to our subconscious, where our ingrained beliefs are held.

In this place, we are more able to let go of limiting beliefs, old habits, and trapped emotions. The depth of our connection allows us to not just live from our mind, but also from our heart. Some experts say the heart sends more messages to the brain than the brain does to the heart. The heart's voice may be our true self, the one that is less analytical and more intuitive. In other words, our heart can guide us to become who we really are.

What does spirituality have to do with becoming who you really are? If we believe that we are a soul, then connection to ourselves and healing ourselves in a deeper way supports becoming who we really are. Our connection to something beyond us can assist us in deepening our love for ourselves, feeling valued and honored, which is necessary for becoming who you really are and believing that you are enough. In fact, this is foundational: if we do not feel fully loved, we will spend our lives trying to achieve this in other ways. Like Sisyphus and the rock, we will keep pushing against something, sometimes ourselves.

What is this divine within and outside of us?

> *I believe there's an intelligence, an invisible conscious-ness within each of us which acts as a giver of life [...] It creates almost 100 trillion specialized cells, starting with only two, and keeps our hearts beating hundreds of thousands times per day. It can organize hundreds of thousands of chemical reactions in a single cell in every second. I reason, if this intelligence is real and is willfully, mindfully, and lovingly demonstrating such amazing abilities, maybe I can take my attention off my external world and begin to go within to develop a relationship with it.*
>
> —*Dr. Joe Dispenza,* You are the Placebo: Making Your Mind Matter.

I invite you to connect more deeply to yourself, as opposed to something outside of you.

Use whatever language you would like to describe the spiritual source: God, The Creator, the Source, or a Higher Self. Whatever you choose, *this* is spirituality. It is all of life, and it is all encompassing.

The spiritual represents the essence of who we are, the exploration of our inner selves at a deeper level, and with that exploration comes the questions. *Who are we? Who else is here? If there is something beyond me or within me, how do I connect to that?* You might also ask yourself, *should I connect with that?* I believe that many women continually ask "Who am I?" and sometimes I believe that this is because we intuitively know that we have been pushing ourselves and allowing society to push us into some one we are not. Deepening into your being-ness, as a divine being, allows you to let go of many of the expectations and issues I have been talking about in this book.

Some people appear to skim the surface of their lives. Simply the fact that you are reading this book and doing this work indicates that you are not a skimmer. You desire depth and are willing to answer the call to do the deep work offered in this book. This call to go within requires facing your shadow beneath the surface, which many of us avoid and hide from. But not you. In religious circles, *un* becoming is often referred to as the dark night of the soul.

What if we could go deeper within? What is possible? This spiritual life I am inviting you to explore is about your *being*, who you truly are beyond your personality. When we go within and connect with others and ourselves this way, we experience moments we can't explain because we are connecting to something beyond us.

I love this statement: *The way out is in.*

The way to become who you really are is from within.

Your being-ness matters.

If Sisyphus was to accept his humanness and go within, what may have been different? Had he been courageous enough to listen and explore living from that place, his eternal struggle may have looked quite different. But how? Sisyphus could have looked within. He could have slowed down, listened, and been guided by his inner knowing. His lack of connection *inward* is one reason he kept focusing *outward*, and from there he could only push and push. He could only see the boulder. Maybe, like many women, he felt empty inside and believed that he needed to do something, so he pushed, gave his power away and simply did what he was told.

One of the greatest travesties of modern society lies in giving our power away. We do this by believing the experts or those who supposedly know what is best for us.

Some believe that we need to go through someone else to connect with the Divine. We don't. Not only do we sometimes think that others know best about spiritual and personal matters for us, but we use God in a way that diminishes us. I used to ask God to tell me what to do about everything. What should I do? Where should I go? When? Then, I came to realize that God doesn't want to direct my life and boss me around. And actually, that's not what I want either. God wants *me* to direct my *own* life and make my own decisions from that inner place of connection to the Divine. That is empowering and freeing, and it is essential for becoming who you really are.

This *un* becoming, this unravelling, is necessary because it allows us to accept the changes and ensuing ups and downs that come with our journey. If we choose to stay in the chaos, to keep pushing our boulders, we recycle a never-ending story of our lives, similar to the story Sisyphus. As Cristen Rodgers put it,

> *Many step foot on the path to spiritual enlightenment expecting it to lead us onward and upward, hoping to become something better than we are, and ready to gather all of the important things we need along the way. What a surprise it is when we eventually realize that this path isn't taking us onward but inward, that we're not gathering things so much as letting them go, and that there was never anything more to aspire to than the truth of what we already are.*

Maybe knowing that you are enough is what being spiritual is all about.

This is why I invite you to explore spirituality. Perhaps this includes noticing and allowing feelings of anger, distrust, dread, or disinterest when this topic arises. Second, it is to invite *you* into your inner world, where I believe that something or some one else dwells within us (God, The Divine, The Creator). Following this path can deepen all the work of this book and perhaps even deepen the belief that you are enough. Third, I invite you to consider and then explore how intuition or your *inner knowing* can be accessed to guide you and help you see yourself fully and clearly.

What Happens When We Over-Focus on Spirituality?

Sometimes, spiritually-focused women will minimize the importance of other aspects of their own being. I've noticed that some women who proclaim they are spiritual, live with a martyr mentality that pushes them to give at the expense of their own health, wellness or even physical needs. As a result, they are poor at self-care, or at setting boundaries. Somehow, the belief that spiritual pursuits are more important than human needs puts a boulder in front of them, and they push. At their own expense.

They may lack connection to their emotions and their inner-knowing and, as a result, their life and service are impeded. Some may put service to others ahead of care and nurture of oneself. They may become tired, exhausted, and physically ill. Spiritual and religious women will sometimes over-emphasize the spiritual life at the expense of the other facets of their human being-ness, not recognizing and accepting that our whole life is a spiritual act. We can become addicted to serving others, the high it brings us, the next person we can help or serve, or the next big idea or pursuit because we need this to feel like we're *enough*. The need to be perfect, to please others, or to over-achieve shows up here. If left unattended, this push to be more and to do more will drive you into this cycle again and again, and it will lead to exhaustion, emptiness, or both. When this happens, notice, love yourself in the midst of your humanity, and make healthier, kinder choices in order to *un* become.

I firmly believe that *un* becoming to become involves addressing your psychological, emotional, physical, and spiritual well-being, and that they are all connected because 'you' are connected. You are one.

Spiritual practice is an invitation to connection, not perfection. Avoid self-judgment (*i.e. Am I doing this right? Am I praying long enough or meditating correctly?*) and allow your humanity, knowing that you will never be perfect and were never meant to be. Maybe part of our *becoming* is accepting our imperfection.

Perfection is not your purpose in life. Becoming you is your purpose in life. Spirituality is the pursuit of connection. Allow, explore, experiment. This is very individual, and it will be unique to you. Having this connection within, to something or someone bigger than yourself, will support you in becoming *you*.

We are a whole being, mind, body, and spirit. The spiritual you *is* your essence, and it is deeply connected to all other parts of you— your mind, your emotions, and your body. In fact, it could be the thread that holds all of 'you' together. What you do to support yourself in one area is also supporting you spiritually, whether you are aware of it or not. For example, some of my women clients who have engaged in the amino acid therapy, often find that their mind is calmer, clearer, and, as a result, their spiritual practices deepen. They can get quiet. They can focus. Those who set boundaries to create more space and time for themselves may find they have more time for spiritual pursuits. Those who let go of the barrage of the inner-critic find that they are more calm, centered, and feel more whole. As you engage in all these ways to support your *un* becoming and becoming, you love yourself more. As you deepen your connection within, you will experience more love and acceptance, which will support your *un* becoming and becoming. Trust yourself to experiment and play with connecting to your inner-self and the Divine within.

Forgiveness Is the Way to Freedom

The act of forgiveness is usually not a one-time endeavor. Forgiveness, in my experience, unfolds. It is a journey. At the same time, it is an intention, a choice, and an act. Much has been written on this elusive topic, however it is through my personal experiences that I have learned how to forgive. Not that I am an expert on doing it, but I have been exploring this and attempting to practice this for a very long time, from both a psychological (human mind) perspective and a spiritual one (divine mind). Forgiveness is an act, not a feeling.

Know that a lack of forgiveness is your way of trying to heal. We hold onto injustices as a way to feel better. But we don't feel better— we feel worse.

I believe that we learn and practice forgiveness through experience: through accepting what has occurred, feeling the emotional impact, and fully allowing our feelings and experience. Without fully feeling, we can't easily forgive and let go. We brush over the pain or the experience and use forgiveness as a way to escape. Without the inner reflection of the real impact on us, we will not be able to release what is there because we have not faced it yet.

Forgiveness is not really about the other person or the wrongdoer. Forgiveness is an act that you alone take on, where you fully face what happened, and you gradually let go of that pain. The focus is on you, not the event or the wrongdoer. You recognize that you no longer want to carry the pain, anger, or hurt, and as you acknowledge these, you choose to start letting go. In this process it is important to focus on you—not the event or the person who you harmed you.

Self-judgment may tell you that you *shouldn't* be angry or hurt, or that you *should* let this go. After all, a good Christian, God follower, or good human *always* forgives. As you *un* become, you will be facing some of these demons—these beliefs that *push* you to forgive too quickly.

Because we want to feel better quickly, we use the concept of forgiveness to push ourselves to fix whatever pain we are experiencing. As the hurt, pain, and betrayal return, keep acknowledging these touch points and allow yourself to gently release what you can, when you can. It takes time.

Forgiveness requires the opposite of pushing. It requires that you allow yourself whatever time you need to weave through forgiveness as an act of self-compassion. Trust that you will know how to let go when the time is right.

What you've been exploring in this book may have given rise to a desire to forgive. It is an act of letting go. Forgiving is courageous because you are letting go of your expectations of the other so you can begin to release the pain that was caused. A lack of forgiveness is usually because of an unmet expectation. (e.g. *They should apologize. They should take accountability. This is not fair. They should not have done this.*) Understanding that we might still be holding onto an expectation is important, but we aren't always aware of what we hold onto. You may need time to determine and be aware of the expectation you are holding. You can't let go of the feeling but you can let go of the expectation, the belief and as you do that, the painful feelings release. A common error women sometimes make is pushing themselves to let go of the feeling. That won't work because as I explained in Chapter 5, on Emotions, feelings are a guidepost. Giving up the need for any expectation is powerfully freeing, *and* it can also be intensely sad. Allow for the sadness and grief as you let go of these expectations and forgive. Offer yourself permission to explore and practice forgiveness without having to do it perfectly.

Forgiving Yourself

Anything that is guilt-inducing is not based in love. This includes the guilt we instill on ourselves when we do not believe that we are measuring up to someone else's standards. Connecting to God or your own higher self should help you feel more loved, supported, and accepted. With this feeling, allow for self-acceptance and the truth that you are enough, and are worthy of compassion. This will help you forgive yourself more compassionately. This will help you see what is beneath the surface and more courageously embrace your whole self. Accepting your shadow and lovingly holding space for both your shadow and your light is a deeply spiritual act.

Forgiving ourselves can be difficult. It bears repeating that we are fundamentally harder on ourselves than we are on others and, as a result, we often hold ourselves to unrealistic standards. We break our promises. We don't live up to our values. We are human, and to be human is to fail. Forgiveness of ourselves involves self compassion, for without being compassionate, our review of what we did or said, or didn't do or say, will come from a place of judgment. Judgment always produces pushing. This will increase our shame. One of the most powerful gifts you can give yourself is forgiveness, but it requires that we face our darkness. Self-compassion will help us do so. The practice of forgiving ourselves also involves giving up expectations, usually the unrealistic ones that we hang on to.

Each time I am faced with the need to forgive, the process and experience is a little different. Each of us will land in judgment and resentment again and again—it is a part of being human. We will also return to forgiveness again and again. This is part of *un* becoming and becoming.

Exercise: A Practice of Forgiveness

As a hypnotherapist, I often use this technique with my clients *and* myself. I will show you how to do this on your own. The main feature of this practice is that it allows you to say anything and everything you want to the other person (without them actually being there physically). Read over these steps first and get comfortable with what the process looks like, then take some uninterrupted time to do this on your own.

1. Close your eyes and begin to relax and notice your breathing. Take your time.

2. When you feel relaxed, allow yourself to see a door. Take in all the details of the door (color, material, size, where the handle is, etc.) and tell yourself that on the other side of the door is your 'healing' room.

3. When you feel ready, move closely to your door, turn the handle, and step into your 'healing room'. Notice two chairs and take a seat in one of them. Invite whoever you want to be in the other chair. Know that they are there to listen and will say nothing. When you are ready, in your mind, begin to tell them anything and everything that you want to say to them, even if you've said it before. Get it all out. Feel the hurt or anger rise and continue to speak or yell at them, in your mind. Swearing may also be an appropriate form of release for you.

4. If you're ready, when you feel you've said everything you want to say, tell them that you forgive them and let them go. If you are not ready to forgive, then don't. Know that you can let them go when you are ready. Whether you've forgiven them or not, allow them to disappear, and bring in a purple light to fill the room, cover you, and fill you. Know that that healing light is cleansing you of the hurt, anger, and grief. that you have been feeling. Know that even if you couldn't forgive, you release a lot and can experience a level of healing.

5. When you are ready leave the room and then open your eyes.

6. Feel free to journal your experience.

Many find that this practice, even it is only done a few times with the same issue or person, has an amazing power to help release what you have been carrying. Sometimes, as you give voice to your needs, emotions arise, anger gives way to hurt, and sometimes tears come. Know that this is healing and as you heal, you are becoming you.

Spirituality Reflections

1. When you think about spirituality, what feelings or thoughts emerge? Allow yourself to be really honest. Have you felt the constraints of religion? Are you wary of rules or judgment about your beliefs?

2. If you're ready to engage in some spiritual practices, what might you do or continue to do? It could be meditation, yoga, prayer, journaling, gatherings, music, worship, etc.

3. What beliefs might you want to let go of so you can connect with your Divine Source, God, Creator, or just yourself within?

4. If you've ever experienced a Divine or spiritual connection, what was that like for you?

5. How might this connection assist in you in believing that you are enough and becoming who you really are?

Spirituality is Both Ordinary and Practical

"The great lesson is that the sacred is in the ordinary, that it is to be found in one's daily life, in one's neighbors, friends and family, in one's backyard."
—Abraham Maslow

It is important to let go of the idea that spirituality is something that is lofty and amazingly deep. Spirituality is also immensely ordinary.

It is in the ordinary of life where you may find the Divine, God, or connection to your true or higher self. In those moments, or in regular, daily activities such as watering the flowers, doing laundry, and creating a meal, you may feel and sense this connection. It may be subtle and quiet, but it is there for you, always.

Many women feel their soul, human essence, and God's presence when they connect with nature and the outdoors. They run. They walk. They forest bathe. They sit by the water. They hug and sit by trees. Letting go of rigid expectations may be freeing.

Also, what time of day is best for you to meditate, pray, slow down, be quiet and sit? When you are engaging in spiritual practices, do you have the sense that you are enough already, or do you attempt to improve yourself?

After fighting with the expectation for most of my life that I should journal, meditate and have quiet time in the morning I have finally accepted that this is not the best time for me. I am wired to plan, so my brain starts thinking and planning when I wake up. For a long time, I resisted this but with little success and quite a lot of self-judgment. I was pushing. I was not accepting my flow. My quiet time is better in the evening. This is when I can reflect and quiet myself to pray, reflect, meditate, journal or engage in self-hypnosis. This is a better rhythm for me. Your rhythm is your rhythm. And what you do for spiritual connection is also you. Remember that the purpose of spiritual practice is to help you connect to your Higher Self, God, The Divine, the Source, the Universe, and yourself.

Exercise: One Way to Practice Connecting Within.

1. Choose a quiet place with uninterrupted time.

2. Have your journal and pen ready to write.

3. Close your eyes and imagine a space within yourself, that inner-most you, where the Divine dwells. Some imagine a healing or sacred room, similar to the room you imagined with the forgive-ness process. First, notice the door, the color of it, the shape and size and the materials it is made of. Then, notice the door handle. Take your time with this. When you are ready, imagine yourself stepping forward, turning the handle, opening the door, and stepping into your sacred space. Take your time and notice what the room looks like, what it feels like. Some notice furniture, some notice Light. Once you feel that you are in this room and have taken in what it looks like, invite your messenger or wisdom giver into your room. Some invite Jesus, some Mother Mary, some simply invite in an important Messenger. Some see themselves when the messenger comes. Some see an angel, or a loved one who has passed. Notice who or what you see. Then, allow yourself to feel, see, or hear a message for you. Some of you may think that you don't see, hear, or feel anything. Trust that you do. It is that still small voice within. You may be more inclined to be more visual, or auditory, or sensory. Allow what you notice to emerge. This may take some time, but you can actually create and enhance this inner sanctuary over time.

4. Whether you feel that you are in that place or not, trust that you are. It isn't important that you get this right, just that you are doing it.

5. Begin to ask questions in your mind and write down both the question and the answer. Allow the answer to flow in from that place within and trust yourself. Allow this to happen for as long as you like, or just be present in the experience. Sometimes, nothing comes to—just a feeling of peace, which is amazingly beautiful.

6. When you're done, thank the Messenger for the connection and allow them to leave the room, knowing that they are always with you.

7. Re-read what you wrote. How does the tone of the answers differ from your questions? Is it different? Is the feeling different? These Messengers are immensely more loving toward you than you are toward yourself.

8. Continue this practice as often as you like. As you deepen your connection to your inner sanctuary over time, you will easily be able to connect here without as much effort. Over time, you will be better able to discern, what is coming from your deep inner-knowing, the Divine, and what is coming from your own mind.

9. The benefits of such a connection are many: more peace, more discernment and intuition about what is right for you and what is not, more confidence, more calm, more acceptance, and more being.

You may also imagine your path of life. As you imagine all the details—the path itself, the sky, the nature, the sounds, the smells—you can imagine a bench on the path. You invite your messenger to join you on the bench. Then, continue in the same way as above allowing your Messenger to be with you and provide a message. Your imagination is endless, so feel free to come up with your own scene.

Finding the Connection Within

Your intuition begins to emerge with more clarity as you *un* become. Once you engage in attention to yourself in a healthy manner, through all the ways I have shared in this book, you begin to free up space and time to be you and to create a more healthful way of living. Another beautiful aspect that starts to emerge for women is an increased experience of intuition. If you are too busy, how can you tune into your inner being? How can you hear if there is too much noise? If you do things that go against your values and overburden yourself with trying to be perfect or to over please people, you won't hear that still, small voice. By engaging in a life that is frenzied and overwhelming, you are actually sending the message to yourself that you don't matter. Your inner self will not trust you to make good decisions about your life. As you start to courageously step out of self-sabotaging and limiting beliefs about yourself, as you *un* become, your sense of self-trust will grow. Trust that you have inner knowing and practice deepening into your intuition.

I've discovered that for the women who want to be their real selves, to *un* become and become, the need to delve into the spiritual realm inevitably comes into play. We simply aren't as effective or fulfilled, even at work, when we separate ourselves into mind *or* body *or* spirit. You are *one*.

One client, who was a very effective and successful leader, hired me for leadership coaching. She wanted to be better. We engaged in a lot of coaching conversations that focused on her leadership role, but it was when her comments shifted to guilt, lack of forgiveness, and feeling disconnected, that the conversation shifted to her spiritual life.

We decided to proceed with a few hypnotherapy sessions. Through these, she released guilt about an abortion, guilt about the belief that she was abandoning her children, guilt that kept her from being free to be herself in both her personal and professional world. In the deepened state of hypnotherapy, she had conversations with those she felt she had let down, including her unborn child. She shared with me that she also felt an overwhelming Love from God in those sessions. She felt it *deeply*. Guilt had disconnected her from God and herself. But she forgave herself. It was intensely personal and power-ful for her.

Questions for Further Reflection on Spirituality

Choose a few questions at a time to reflect on. You can always come back to other questions later.

1. What do you think about the statement that all of life is spiritual? What might that mean to you?

2. What do you think about the notion that integrating all of the information in this book into your own life is a spiritual act?

3. What do you notice about your thoughts or beliefs when you begin to think about spirituality?

4. What has been your experience of forgiving others?

5. What might you be open to, going forward? Forgiveness? Journaling? Meditation? Prayer? Anything else considered spiritual? If it's nothing, honor that. Rest is spiritual.

6. If you've been part of a religious group that instilled more fear, or even judgment, than love, what have you done to move away from that self judgment? It can be difficult to unravel the *shoulds* and the *dos* from these experiences. Sometimes, there is fear in stepping away from a group or long-held beliefs—fear that you've failed God or others, that you are being disobedient. It's immensely courageous to step away, however this may be exactly what you've needed in order to *become you.*

7. If you connect within yourself and begin to trust your inner knowing in a deeper way, what might change for you? What might you start doing to enhance your awareness of and trust in your inner knowing?

Creativity

Creative endeavors assist with the journey inward, with connecting to the parts of you that have not been attended to or that feel separate from one another. Creativity has the potential to bypass our conscious mind, allowing us to be *less thinky* and more in *flow*. So, this is an important piece in becoming *you*. In fact, creativity is incredibly healing, and it can help us let go of what is not us, our *un* becoming. I believe that women are incredibly creative beings, but we often abandon creative pursuits in favour of people and projects that we believe are more important.

We desire creativity but we don't do it. Most if not all women I know, (myself included) speak about wanting to quilt, sew, draw, paint, garden, learn calligraphy, take an art class, learn to make jewelry, or pursue other creative endeavors, but we rarely or never take the time to do these things. They just don't seem purposeful enough.

What if creating actually helped support you in *un* becoming and becoming by nourishing and spending time with your inner self?

Questions for Reflection

1. What do you do, or have you done in the past that you consider creative? Here are some examples: colouring, painting, journaling, dancing, singing, gardening, writing, day-dreaming.

2. When you engaged in this activity without any expectation, but with the pure freedom to just *create*, how did you feel? Describe this. Feel free to even sketch this feeling. Take a few moments to draw, doodle, or color your creative expression of this feeling or this experience.

3. What did you love doing creatively when you were a kid? How did you feel at those times?

4. How might creativity help you *un* become what isn't you and help you become who you really are?

5. What might you need to let go of? What beliefs might you need to let go of? For me, the belief that I have to produce, gets in the way of me creating. I often tussle with this idea that I must always be productive and do something meaningful. This is one of my pushes. Another one of my pushes is that I don't think I'm very good at art, so I don't like to do it. It's my self judging that gets in the way. What I have discovered is that I like to write, journal and play with poetry. This is more me and is actually healing and nourishing.

6. What form of creativity is more you?

7. What might you start doing, even in a small way that might be a creative practice for you?

Creative Playdate Exercise

The intention behind this exercise is to use creativity to connect with yourself, to be 'with' you. That's it. A playdate with yourself. It's simple: make a date with yourself in the next week. This is for you, and you alone. Carve out and schedule at least one hour. Think ahead of something creative you would like to try, and even experiment with. Maybe you have been wanting to try watercolor painting, sketching with charcoals, writing poetry, dancing, calligraphy, or maybe even a vision board. Maybe you want to colour. It may be something you loved doing in the past but haven't done in a while. It might be something brand new. Choose one idea and plan ahead by gathering the materials so you are ready for your creative playdate.

Try to approach it with open-heartedness. Notice any resistance that may arise. Allow it.

Follow These Steps:

1. Schedule the time.

2. Plan ahead and choose one thing to do.

3. Gather the supplies ahead of time.

4. Protect this creative play date with yourself.

5. Ahead of time, imagine feeling joy and delight during your playdate.

6. Engage in the creative activity with awareness and mindfulness. In other words, try to be in the moment. Notice any judgment or frustrations. Be with them and allow them to pass.

7. Following your creative playdate, take time to journal your experience. Perhaps you will notice some self-judgment. (*I'm not good at this. I'm not creative.*) Journal what felt good and right about this experience, too.

Moving Forward

I'm a person who tries to fit things together, to integrate things, to see how parts fit. So, it's no wonder that I've been intrigued by spirituality and knowledge. Part of the purpose of this book is to help you, the reader, explore how all of this connects within you. Connecting with myself was deeply valuable to me and as I did, my beliefs about God and spiritual truth, among other things, shifted and became more meaningful. I stopped asking what to do and started following my intuition and heart more. My beliefs about God continues to transform to this day. This means that I may continue to question who

God or the Divine is. What role does this Being play in my life? At times, I'm not even sure what to call this Being, but I feel and experience the connection more deeply as I continue to *un* become because I am becoming much more accepting of who I am, my shadow and my light. I think that my most profound *un* becoming was letting go of the notion that I had to understand who or what God is.

This may be uncomfortable for some, but for others this may provide freedom.

Your journey is your journey, and how you interpret this chapter is completely up to you. If you accept parts or reject all of it, that's great, because *you* are choosing and deciding what is best for *you*. My intent here is to offer some insights and to share some of my story to invite you to explore your spiritual path and beliefs with openness and curiosity.

Thank you for listening.

You are enough.

Chapter Thirteen

Becoming 'You': Putting It All Together

"Though no one can go back and make a brand new start,
anyone can start from now and make a brand new ending."
—Carl Bard

Let's circle back: Imagine a world where women are powerful and strong. A world where women know that they are enough, and they live and serve from their enough-ness. A world where women live life, fully free to be who are. This is you! This is who you are becoming!

The integration of all this information happens by understanding it, assessing yourself, doing it and, lastly, being it. You become who you really are with all of these pieces.

Can We Talk?

I know this information is life-changing because I needed it, and I've done it. Every. Single. Piece. I was able to become more of who I really am when I gave myself the time and practice to do all the things I talk about in this book. I couldn't do it all at once, but that is part of the process. I had to do it a bit at a time. I am always becoming more me. These pieces that I share in this book did not come to me in a linear fashion, much of it overlapped and interrelated all along my journey.

I had to understand that I had forgotten how to say, or had never ever learned to say, "Stop. This is too much. This is too much work, and too much doing, and too much responsibility. I can't do it all." I was overly responsible.

In other words, my first big 'Aha!' was that I desperately needed to set boundaries to become who I really am. I was in my twenties, and I was really stuck between pleasing others and setting boundaries. As I tied it together, I slowly began to walk out of the bleakness and the stuckness that I had created. For some reason I can't explain, it was crucial for me to know why I hadn't been setting boundaries. Once I had that piece of information, knowing I was invested in pleasing others and being an over-achiever, I could begin the work of changing the beliefs I had about myself, thereby un becoming these entangled beliefs and behaviours.

The 'I am enough' statement didn't come until much later, but at some level, even back then, I was working on believing that I had inherent value. Eventually, all of this reflecting led me to sort out that my being-ness impacted my doing, and if I didn't value myself, I would use other people or activities to make me feel better about 'me'. Over-achieving and over-pleasing gave me a false sense of value. Even when I understood that I was doing this, it still took me a long time to walk out from under the power of those limiting beliefs. In fact, it took years—yes, even decades—and I am still walking out of it. Every. Single. Day.

When I started practicing psychology, I began to add the emotional work to my life and my clients. I saw how accepting my feelings was crucial to my mental, emotional, and even physical health. I made a personal practice of this and learned much from thousands of conversations. I was astounded by how this work affected the women I was working with. They spoke of how free they felt when they began to accept their feelings, without judgment. This was a critical shift for me. And was freeing. This became my go to, my primary focus and it still is.

This long and winding journey to un become informed my spiritual journey, too. A deepening spiritual connection helped me move through my stuff, sometimes bringing awareness to my self-judgment, helping me forgive and let go, helping me accept myself more fully, and all these threads came together into one theme—becoming who I really am. Spirituality was part of my journey to becoming, from the beginning and was with me all along the way.

Another thread to arrive was how un becoming related to other people. This was not a smooth ride. I have many and varied relationships, both supportive and challenging, where un becoming taught me even more about who I am. Relationships challenged my boundaries, strengthened my ability to ask for what I need, and in some cases, taught me to let go.

All of these threads were part of the boulder that I had been pushing up my own mountain. Allowing my emotions to exist without judgement helped me push less against myself. In my early years, I didn't use the term self-care. but this is what I was doing by paying attention to how I felt. I listened to my body, I noticed what I was feeling and decided to do less when I was tired or overwhelmed. And I am still learning this.

Sometimes, I felt guilty and thought I was lazy when my body was not responding the way I thought it should be. I lived in exhaustion for a couple of decades. As I kept re-establishing boundaries and stepping back, I made choices to honor my time, which honored me. This helped, but it didn't help me feel healthy or energetic. I found work, tasks, and conversations emotionally draining. I limited my work to three days a week to try to cope, but I still didn't feel better. That's when my pursuit and practice of brain health nutrition came in.

These natural and alternative healing approaches helped me to overcome my insomnia, and my energy improved. After that, at least I was sleeping. Up until that time, no amount of sleep brought me rest or pulled me out of exhaustion, yet this did. It also resolved some of my anxiety and low-grade depression. The truth is, I had experienced this for most of my life but hadn't paid much attention to it. I was even on an antidepressant for a few years, and while they helped, this brain health piece was the missing piece in my healing journey.

Then, the science of happiness and the power of the mind became of interest to me, and I began to practice and experiment with various techniques. These additional resources allowed me to feel even better physically, emotionally, and mentally—and maybe spiritually as well! My busy, cluttered mind made meditation, prayer, and slowing down almost impossible. Yet, all of these pieces have helped me create a more confident belief in myself. I forged ahead, took business risks, and put myself out there. It was painful, and self-doubt would often creep in, leaving me to feel awful about myself. Those doubts are fewer now. I am much more accepting of myself.

The last piece I incorporated was self-compassion. Interestingly, the piece I believe to be foundational, I incorporated last. By the time I got here, my health was much better, my mind was calmer, my confidence had grown, and my brain time was not consumed with worry, over-thinking, and planning. But, self-compassion! Wow! It's so simple, yet so profound. It was like finding fifth gear when I'd been driving in fourth. Things may have been good, but fifth gear accelerated me to becoming a more healthy and whole version of myself. I think it's my favorite tool, now and although I wasn't aware of the term 'self compassion' before, all the work I was doing—like being less judgmental of myself, tuning into my body, allowing myself to feel what I felt, etc.—were self-compassionate acts. So, the groundwork had been laid.

All these threads are how I continue to become who I really am. I continue to unravel, deepen, and change my thoughts and beliefs, which profoundly impact my choices and behaviours. Each thread is part of the tapestry of becoming me.

I am learning that 'I am enough'.

Final Thoughts

The journey to become who you really are is not for the weak of heart. The courage to *un* become means looking within, changing thoughts, and choosing new behaviours. It means giving up on pushing the boulder.

It means going into your darkness and being willing to embrace your shadow. It means giving up who you were, and perhaps even the life you created. But the magic is on the other side, and as you become *you* and now you are free to express more of the real you, to the world.

Sisyphus never stopped pushing. As far as we know, he never paused to reflect on his situation or his journey. You, however, have stopped pushing. Not always, but sometimes—and that's enough. You have paused. You have reflected on your rock and why you pushed it. The rock might never disintegrate, but you are now conscious of it, you can step around it, you can choose to stop fighting it. You can do better because now you know better.

Know this. Know that whenever you feel overwhelmed, whenever life is unravelling and your heart hurts deeply, or whenever the loss is so great and you're feeling alone, this happens to many of us. Life includes pain and loss, and it will feel too great to bear at times. Make a promise to yourself to always come back to how you feel and to support yourself with self-compassion. This will cut through the mind chatter.

The journey of *un* becoming can feel like a total undoing at times. It will hurt, it will be hard, and it will take courage.

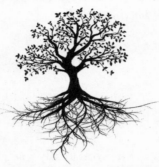

"Inside every seed is the DNA of an entire tree, and the blueprint of a forest that will grow out of it. You are a seed. You do not 'have' what it takes to fulfill your purpose. 'You' are what it takes."
—Jordon Veira

Your journey, your process of *un* becoming who you created yourself to be, to become the *real* you, involves recognizing that you've always been there. Becoming *you* is not about perfection, dear traveller. It is about uncovering what may have been there all this time and nurturing that *you* to be *you*. You are that seed, and in order to be the real you, you've had to let go of what no longer serves you, like when dead wood and old branches and overgrowth are pruned from a tree. Remember, when dead wood and overgrowth is pruned, the tree grows stronger. Letting go of what is not *you* is painful, but necessary. Becoming you makes that *you* stronger.

We are human and the process of integrating all of you is never done. Your becoming is never done.

The difference is that now, you are more able to manage setbacks because you've learned to be more self-compassionately supportive of yourself. You'll be softer and kinder toward yourself and others. You're more able to allow feelings to rise, to hold them, and be with them. You're becoming more courageous in setting boundaries and saying "no" to what is not good for you, and you're even becoming courageous in saying no to what is not the best for you. It's the lack of acceptance of yourself and your suffering that causes you a great deal of pain. So, going forward, know your vulnerabilities and prepare for them. You will have setbacks. I do. We all do.

So, you may never be done with this book. I invite you to return to any chapter to revisit a topic that you want to focus on or understand more fully. Like I said, I always return to self-compassion. I never stop being aware of my stress levels or working at being clear with others about my "no" and my "yes." I am always cognizant of my own boundaries, and I use the amino acid therapy approach as well as brain practices to take care of my brain. All of this forms the foundation for how I treat and feel about myself.

Reflecting on Your Journey

Well done! You've reached the end of this book, but this is not the end. Actually, there is no end to your becoming, which means life can only deepen and get better from here.

Let's take some time to honor you and all you have done in this past while:

No matter how much you think you did or didn't do with the concepts in this book, you did some work. What has the process of *un* becoming felt like for you?

Take your time with these reflection questions as you are reviewing the concepts you have engaged with so far. Do one question at a time and sit with it awhile if you like, then move on to the next. Remember to be compassionate and accepting toward yourself as you review and reflect.

1. As you've engaged in self-care, what are you noticing about guilt? Self-judgment? Your energy? Your mind? Your sleep?

2. Review the past few months: limiting beliefs, self-compassion, boundaries, emotions, courageous connections, and self-care. What have been the most impactful concepts for you? How so?

3. If you've been thinking about how all of this impacts you at work, in your business, or in your leadership role, how might self-compassion, boundaries, and letting go of your limiting beliefs assist you at work?

4. Where have you made the most meaningful change in your life? What has been the impact of this on you and on others in your personal and/or professional life? What are you most proud of?

A Plan for Going Forward

Questions for Reflection: What do you need in order to continue your personal and professional growth? Do you need mentoring? Coaching? Workshops or courses? Reading? Other resources, like meeting regularly with a friend or a group of friends? We all need accountability such as a trusted and supportive thought partner, to help us continue to become. Create and write out your go forward plan that will support your continued work in *un* becoming and becoming you. Some of the tips to follow will help you.

Exercise: What three practices are you willing to commit to in order to go forward? How will you keep doing them? What do you need?

When you focus on a few small things, the big things change. The smallest things can create the biggest change. The magic is in the repetition. If you take just a few concepts from this workbook and focus on understanding yourself and taking action with them, you will ignite a ripple effect which will bring you closer to becoming *you*. Work through one area to get the change anchored. Get your new habits in place, and then move on to the next.

Some Additional Help: What Creates Success?

Try these simple things:

1. Commit to practicing self-care on a daily basis.

2. Take responsibility by letting go of shaming and blaming yourself and others.

3. Be kinder to yourself and continue to anchor into self-compassion as the heartbeat that keeps everything alive.

4. Focus on the first few things you feel compelled to work on, such as boundaries, assertiveness, brain nutrition, or positivity. Other concepts are important but focus on one or two of these and the others will follow.

5. Get support. Continue to connect with other women, friends or colleagues, a counsellor, or a coach. Remember, you can't become *you* alone. Talk, share, and practice vulnerability.

6. Remember that *un* becoming and becoming take time. In fact, it will be your journey for your whole life. As much as you recall, practice patience as you strengthen the belief that you are enough.

7. What else should be on this list? What would you add that works for you?

"He said, 'You become. It takes a long time. That's why it doesn't happen often to people who break easily, or have sharp edges, or who have to be carefully kept. Generally, by the time you are Real, most of your hair has been loved off, and your eyes drop out and you get loose in the joints and very shabby. But these things don't matter at all, because once you are Real, you can't be ugly, except to people who don't understand."
—The Velveteen Rabbit

You are enough.
You were always enough.
You will always be enough.

Appendix

This book is part workbook, part theory, and part story. It's designed to provide a step-by-step roadmap for your journey toward *becoming*, but there is no "right" way to use this book. Here are some ideas:

Work Through this Book with a Group of Women

Gather a group of like-minded, open-hearted, and soul-centered women to discuss and support the unfolding changes in each of your lives as you work through this process. Read one chapter at a time and complete the exercises and questions. Then, meet to discuss the content, your answers to the questions, and your experiences, one chapter at a time. Take your time. You are worth it. Your life is not a race. It is a journey. You're not behind. You are enough.

Deep, personal work and growth is always enriched when you are supported. Everything you need is here. Whatever group you are a part of—spiritual, church groups, healing circles, women's groups, and more—will benefit.

I suggest forming a group of eight women or less, who meet every two to four weeks for ninety minutes at a time. Some chapters may require more time than others. Gather your group, write, record, and share what is happening and how you are changing. Share your courageous actions. Women supporting women is powerful, necessary, and magical. Group work creates an experience of being known and connected. Thoughts and experiences are validated which allows for an opportunity of self-acceptance.

Through discussion, exercises, self-coaching, accountability and support, your personal and/or professional growth builds on each chapter you work on. You can share your experiences and have an opportunity to hear other's stories. You will enter into the lives of others at a deep level and allow others into your world in the same way. Connecting with other women helps us connect to ourselves. Working in isolation is rarely effective. We need to know that we are accepted and loved as we navigate personal change. This supportive, non-judgmental group connection helps support our enough-ness through the chaos that can ensue when we try to affect change on our own.

To get you started, consider using this simple structure.

1. **First Meeting:**

   a. Review the book prior to meeting so you have an overview of the content.

   b. Confirm how often you want to meet, for how long, and when. I recommend at least a two-week gap (perhaps more) in between gatherings. Let your group decide what works best. The time in between allows you time to read the chapter, answer the questions, do the exercises, and begin to implement the content into your life.

   c. Review homework for the next meeting. In preparation for your second meeting, the homework would be to read the first chapter, answer the questions, do the exercises, and begin to implement and practice the concepts into your life. If you can, work through chapter one on your own. This is why you may only meet every 3- 4 weeks. It takes time to review the chapter, complete the exercises, journal and then begin to create new changes in your life.

d. Share why you are working through this book and what you hope to get out of it.

e. To keep the group running smoothly, create some rules of engagement. (See example below.) These may include turning cell phones off, starting and ending on time, coming prepared, or a procedure in the event that someone is late or does not come prepared. Make sure to identify who holds who accountable. Once the rules are agreed to, have someone write them up and send them out to each participant.

f. Review your agreement (on the following page) prior to your second meeting. Note: this agreement is a commitment to yourself and to the group, and it must include a confidentiality statement to maintain an experience of personal safety.

g. You may want to create an online private group where you can ask questions of each other and share challenges and successes between meetings. Confirm who will set this up and who will be the moderator. This helps build connections with one another and can provide additional support and accountability.

2. **Second Meeting and Beyond**

a. Prior to any gathering, read through the appropriate chapter on your own and complete the questions and exercises. Decide how many or which ones you are committed to finishing. Come prepared to share insights and experiences with your group.

b. Consider starting each session with a question, such as "What went well these past few weeks?" to check-in. Consider giving each person three minutes to respond to keep things moving.

c. On week two, review the rules of engagement and make any changes necessary.

d. Have each person share their experience with the material from that week's chapter.

e. Review any homework.

f. Go through some of the questions in the chapter. Remember, it's okay not to get to all of them. Allow each person a chance to share their answer.

g. Share experiences with any of the exercises.

h. Share what action you will take for the next few weeks.

i. As self-care is a fundamental component to *un* becoming to become, I encourage you to regularly ask *what am I doing for self-care this week?*

j. Take turns leading.

3. **Conclusion of Group**

a. Identify up to three areas that you are committed to addressing as you move forward, and how you will do that. (For example, boundaries, self-compassion, courageous conversations, brain health, spirituality, etc.)

b. As you come to the close of the book, you may wish to continue meeting as a group, or take a break and then resume. If you continue meeting, decide what content you want to revisit.

Example: Becoming *You* Group Agreement
and/or Individual Agreement:

Please do your best to commit to the exercises and homework in between your meeting times before you move on to the next chapter. These have been designed to help you reflect, grow, and become you. It is important to reflect on one chapter at a time and then create some action before moving onto the next.

- Your full participation in our meetings is encouraged and expected. It will assist you in becoming *you*, and it will assist other women in becoming them.

- The facilitator's role (if there is one) is to encourage group discussion through coaching and questions.

- The goal for you as the participant is to have an opportunity to talk about what you are learning and how it is being integrated into your life as you continue to gain insight into your beliefs and behaviours, always moving closer to the real you. It is also important to share any challenges.

- Understanding, reflection, and then action are foundational to this process.

- In order to focus on the session and keep to a timely schedule, we commit to equal time for all. If someone is interested in a more thorough discussion and time does not permit, we encourage the individual to discuss this with her mentor, friend, and/or the group facilitator.

- Refrain from offering advice unless asked. Focus on you. If someone asks for advice, a good rule of thumb is to turn it around and ask them what they think.

- Your investment in these sessions will have a direct impact on what you receive. You are encouraged to attend all sessions prepared, to complete homework in between sessions and to share and discuss.

Note: Becoming You Book Clubs

- Please feel free to reach out to me (w.tl@sasktel.net) to let me know you are hosting a book club.

- Please post photos of your group/club, tag Wendy Turner-Larsen and #becomingyouforwomen

Becoming *You*: Goals & Development Plan

Name: _____

Date: _____

Vision Statement: Who am I? What are some of my unique gifts which I bring to, or express in the world?

_____

_____

Development Goal #1:

_____

Specific Steps:

   1. _____

      • _____ (Sub steps)

- _____
- _____

2. _____

3. _____

Development Goal #2:

_____

Specific Steps:

1. _____

2. _____

3. _____

Who Else Can Use this Book

If you are a health coach, counsellor, psychologist or healing professional serving others, consider using this book with your clients to help them reflect, change, and grow. Read and work through one chapter at a time or have them read the entire book and then go back and process more deeply. When I was a psychologist in private practice, I often recommended books to my clients and suggested they read a chapter and then journal their thoughts about it. Many found themselves unable to journal without guidance. This book can support that practice.

If you are a human resource professional, create mastermind groups, accountability groups, and power circles to utilize *un*-becoming to ignite and grow women leaders and team members.

If you are a senior leader, you may also want to consider mastermind groups with your peers. You could also use this book as a mentorship path for upcoming leaders. Personal development promotes a greater sense of confidence, courage, and resilience in young women leaders.

I run a program supporting women leaders as they work on the personal side of their lives to transform their leadership. I find that they experience greater calm, and they are more focused, more present with their employees, and are more creative and productive as they *un* become. Self-doubt and imposter syndrome can be a huge saboteur for a leader who wants to be authentic, lead from a place of wholeness, and be truly impactful. The old paradigm of be-more and do-more in leadership is exhausting women leaders.

If you are an executive or leadership coach, consider using this book with your clients to create greater self-awareness, enhance confidence, address the root of limiting beliefs and behaviours, and increase self-care and resilience. You may also find the chapter on Emotions helpful for your clients. Many leaders struggle with a lack of confidence or self-doubt. It is usually lurking somewhere, and it gets in the way. The limiting beliefs and stress assessments may also be helpful.

Many leaders feel they that don't have enough time to do everything they need to do to be a successful leader. This book helps clear the clutter so leaders can focus on what is truly important and move forward from a place of calm centeredness instead of frenzied activity. *Un*-becoming can help your clients understand the root of their self-sabotaging behaviours and shift it to a more positive place. The questions, exercises, and resources are here to assist their process of transformation.

If you are an educator or teacher, you may want to create groups for girls and young women. The key is the material, the questions, the exercises, the homework, the discussion and the support of others.

Self-Care List

The act of self-care is powerful. Shifting attention to yourself creates a change in your mindset which sends a message to your brain that you matter. Below you will find a list of self-care practices to support you. As you use them, I encourage you to practice being mindful and in the moment. Your mind might wander, but the act of putting attention on yourself for a few minutes every day will change you.

Write out 20 things you like to do or would like to explore for self-care. These should be enjoyable for you. This can feel challenging, which is why I included it here. It's not an extra. It's essential. Here are some ideas:

- Review your three-word mantra about yourself, and say it regularly—*I am kind, I am strong, I am loved.*
- Practice the visualization exercise at the end of Chapter Four— Limiting Beliefs
- Create a spiritual practice
- Engage with your creativity
- Have a leisurely cup of tea without distractions
- Take a fifteen-minute break and do nothing
- Take a walk outside
- Grow a garden
- Craft (knitting, scrapbooking, photography, sewing, etc.)
- Take your camera/phone outside and photograph what you love
- Take a bath
- Read your favourite book
- Daydream
- Meditate
- Pray
- Write in your journal

- Enjoy coffee or lunch with a friend
- Book a massage
- Join in a sport or activity you love (running, kayaking, canoeing)
- Play a boardgame with a family member
- Give or receive a back rub/foot rub
- Purchase new bedsheets and curl up for an afternoon reading
- Buy a new book or go borrow one from the library
- Buy a daily reading book
- Write down ten things you are grateful for
- Walk your dog
- Pet your cat
- Any or all of the Big Three brain exercises
- Do the meditation on connecting within in Chapter Twelve—Creativity & Spirituality
- What do you like to do for self-care?

Further Resources on Brain Health and Nutrition

Now that you've completed the Four-Part Mood Type Questionnaire and read through the explanation of the neurotransmitters, related symptoms, and the positive outcomes, consider exploring other resources.

How to address depleted brain chemistry with Amino Acid Therapy and other neuronutrients (natural supplements):

1. Purchase and review the book, *The Mood Cure* by Julia Ross. This is a two-part treatment regimen. The first part describes the use of specific amino acids and other supplements to address false moods caused by neurotransmitter depletion. The second part of this book is food based (in addition to an exploration of other

supporting supplements and an exploration of adrenal fatigue and thyroid dysfunction). It's important to learn to eat in a way that nourishes and supports your brain chemistry. The Four-Part Mood Type Questionnaire (at the beginning of Chapter Ten) will help guide you. You can also refer to www.moodcure.com for articles, information, and more resources.

2. Be vigilant in following the guidelines in *The Mood Cure* if you choose to do this on your own, especially if you have medical or health issues, are pregnant, and/or are presently taking any medication. These precautions are outlined in *The Mood Cure*, and they are for your safety. Pregnant or nursing women are not advised to take the amino acids. If you are on any antidepressants or anti-anxiety medications, please work with a trained practitioner.

3. Check with your doctor and/or pharmacist for any contraindications before you take any of the recommended supplements.

4. Find and work with a practitioner. You can find an expert here: www.moodcure.com

Journaling Suggestions

Use these at any time, or when you run out of journaling ideas:

1. I could gently move from where I am toward where I want to be by choosing ... differently.

2. A self-nurturing activity I enjoy is .....

3. One life insight or word I could choose is .....

4. To be kinder and gentler to myself at work, I will .....

5. An area of my life I can ask for help in is ..... (i.e. work, tasks, emotional support, acknowledgement, etc.)

6. As I review my week, I feel really proud of how I .....

7. When I consider my relationships, I would like to deepen my relationship with ..... by.....

8. I would like to deepen my connection to myself by.....

9. Who do I want to encourage today by paying forward a compliment or acknowledgment?

10. Today the difference between 'being' and 'doing' feels like .....

Books—Resources to Support Your Becoming

The Mood Cure by Julia Ross

Essentials of Managing Stress by Brian Luke Seaward

The Craving Cure by Julia Ross

Attitudes of Gratitude by M. J. Ryan

Boundaries by Dr, Henry Cloud and Dr. John Townsend

Women's Bodies, Women's Wisdom—Christiane Northrup, M.D.

Hardwiring Happiness by Rick Hanson, PhD

Emotional SMARTS by Dr. June Donaldson

Other Tools

Videos

I have created and recorded many videos related to the topics in this book. You can find these on my Facebook Page, Turner Larsen Consulting known as Sense and Soul Saturday.

Facebook Group Becoming You for Women.

I have created a private Facebook Group for women like you that want to be in community with other women as you *un* become and become. Feel free to request to join.

Websites

www.self-compassion.org

www.turner-larsen.com

Retreats, Workshops, and Power Circle Groups—www.turnerlarsen.com

Becoming You for Women—Two Day Workshop

Becoming You for Women—Power Circle Group

Becoming You for Women—Hypnotherapy Groups

Personal/Brain Health/Leadership Coaching

Brain Health Coaching:

www.turnerlarsen.com

www.moodcure.com

Weight Loss with the Brain Health Approach

www.juliarosscures.com

Leadership/Brain/Transformational Coaching:

www.turnerlarsen.com

Counseling/Psychotherapy:

Ask a trusted friend or family member for a counsellor/psychologist recommendation.

Check with your EFAP (Employee and Family Assistance Program through your work, if you have one) coordinator for an approved therapist/counsellor/psychologist in your area.

Check with your insurance company to inquire about approved counsellors/psychologists.

References

Velvet Elvis (2005, 2012)—Rob Bell

Women's Bodies, Women's Wisdom (1994, 1998, 2006)—Dr. Christiane Northrup

Co-Active Coaching: New Skills for Coaching People Toward Success in Work and Life (1998)—Laura Whitworth

The Female Brain (2007)—Dr. Louanne Brizendine, M.D.

The Mood Cure (2002)—Julia Ross

Depression-Free Naturally (2001)—Dr. Joan Matthews Larson, PhD

Seven Weeks to Sobriety (1997)—Dr. Joan Matthews Larson, PhD

You are the Placebo: Making Your Mind Matter (2015)—Dr. Joe Dispenza

Hardwiring Happiness (2013)—Dr. Rick Hanson, PhD

E-Cubed: Nine More Energy Experiments that Prove Manifesting Magic and Miracles is Your Full-Time Gig (2014)—Pam Grout

The Emotional Life of Your Brain (2012)—Dr. Richard Davidson, PhD

The Brain that Changes Itself (2007)—Dr. Norman Doidge, MD

"How Expressing Gratitude Might Change Your Brain"—Christian Jarrett—The Cut—January 7, 2016

"Gratitude and the Brain"—Dr. Daniel Amen—amenclinics.com

The Velveteen Rabbit (1958)—Margery Williams

Note: The recommendations within do not include any medical advice, medical interventions, or diagnosis of any kind. For medical advice, consult your health care professional. For psychological or mental health support, consult a registered psychologist or professional counsellor.

As explained, you are free to work through this book in groups and facilitate discussion as outlined.

This does not include permission to 'teach' this material, without written permission of Wendy Turner-Larsen, w.tl@sasktel.net

About the Author

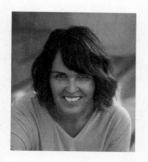

No one could be better placed to write about the process of becoming than Wendy Turner-Larsen. She is a professional coach, workshop facilitator, professional public speaker, and brain nutritionist who has decades of experience as a professional psychologist, counsellor, and spiritual pastor. She has an MA in Counselling/Psychology, an MA in Adult Education, and an MSc in Health and Nutrition Education, as well as several certifications in fields such as neuronutrient therapy and hypnotherapy. The insights in *Becoming 'You' for Women* have formed the basis of her workshops and women's coaching groups as well as the one-on-one counsel she has given to hundreds of women throughout her career.

Turner-Larsen believes that true change can only come about through deep, inner work—that's why she applies all of her teachings to herself first. She is passionate about being healthy—emotionally, mentally, and spiritually—and she strives to share her insights to create deep, lasting change in women. Most importantly, she wrote this book because these concepts work. Turner-Larsen infuses her writing with the knowledge of someone who has already walked this path. Now, she extends a hand to help new travellers find the way.

She currently lives in Regina, Saskatchewan, with her husband.

More information about Wendy Turner-Larsen, her business, and her writing projects can be found on her website: turnerlarsen.com.